AF896621

Eyelid and Conjunctival Tumors

Mathilde Kaspi • Elisa Cinotti
Jean-Luc Perrot • Thibaud Garcin
Editors

Eyelid and Conjunctival Tumors

In Vivo Confocal Microscopy

Springer

Editors
Mathilde Kaspi
Department of Ophthalmology
Centre Hospitalier Universitaire de Saint-Etienne
Loire
France

Elisa Cinotti
Department of Dermatology
University of Siena, S. Maria alle Scotte Hospital
Siena
Italy

Jean-Luc Perrot
Department of Dermatology
Centre Hospitalier Universitaire de Saint-Etienne
Loire
France

Thibaud Garcin
Department of Ophthalmology
Centre Hospitalier Universitaire de Saint-Etienne
Loire
France

ISBN 978-3-030-36605-6 ISBN 978-3-030-36606-3 (eBook)
https://doi.org/10.1007/978-3-030-36606-3

© Springer Nature Switzerland AG 2020
This work is subject to copyright. All rights are reserved by the Publisher, whether the whole or part of the material is concerned, specifically the rights of translation, reprinting, reuse of illustrations, recitation, broadcasting, reproduction on microfilms or in any other physical way, and transmission or information storage and retrieval, electronic adaptation, computer software, or by similar or dissimilar methodology now known or hereafter developed.
The use of general descriptive names, registered names, trademarks, service marks, etc. in this publication does not imply, even in the absence of a specific statement, that such names are exempt from the relevant protective laws and regulations and therefore free for general use.
The publisher, the authors, and the editors are safe to assume that the advice and information in this book are believed to be true and accurate at the date of publication. Neither the publisher nor the authors or the editors give a warranty, expressed or implied, with respect to the material contained herein or for any errors or omissions that may have been made. The publisher remains neutral with regard to jurisdictional claims in published maps and institutional affiliations.

This Springer imprint is published by the registered company Springer Nature Switzerland AG
The registered company address is: Gewerbestrasse 11, 6330 Cham, Switzerland

Preface

It was natural for us to state the two questions that preceded the genesis of this book and that the reader, too, is entitled to ask himself before acquiring and reading this book.

Why two of the co-editors of this book that deals with an ophthalmological area are dermatologists?

What exactly is the part of the ocular system explored in this book and what is the contribution of in vivo confocal microscopy to the study of this area?

We will answer the last question first for the purpose of clarity.

This book studies that part of the ocular system, which we will define as anterior, i.e. all the ocular structures with immediate access to the simple inspection of the eye and the touch, a definition that is more dermatological than ophthalmological.

This, in our opinion, is what makes this book so original because this part of the eye is on the border between dermatology and ophthalmology.

Although there are already magnificent books on confocal microscopy in ophthalmology, they focus on the cornea and the adjacent limbic region. However, the contribution of the dermatological practice and of skin-specific imaging techniques allowed us to examine the whole anterior part of the eye.

Being not attached to a support, our confocal microscopy camera dedicated to dermatology offered us the possibility to explore the first 300–800 microns of all the different parts constituting the anterior ocular system (conjunctiva, eyelid and cornea) *in vivo* and at the microscopic scale. Confocal microscopy cameras dedicated to ophthalmology cannot access all these areas for purely mechanical reasons (because they are fixed on a support).

Most of our images have been acquired in reflectance mode, and only few in the fluorescence mode which is a research approach for the moment.

Why was this book co-written by dermatologists and ophthalmologists?

This book is the iconographic summary of 7 years of dermato-ophthalmological multidisciplinary consultations of confocal microscopy concerning any lesions of the anterior ocular system.

We wanted to share the richness of the iconography accumulated during this period as well as the experience acquired. The recruitment of our patients also derived both from dermatology and ophthalmology consultations. We had the audacity to make this hybrid medical book of dermatology and ophthalmology imaging. This book seemed to us to reflect the medical mutation that new imaging techniques and more particularly confocal microscopy cause.

The images form the framework of this book. These are many confocal microscopy images of course but also anatomopathological sections of the different tumors presented. It should always be borne in mind that the interpretation of confocal microscopy images is based on anatomopathology. Confocal microscopy is not intended to replace anatomopathology, but on the contrary is based on it.

We wanted ophthalmologists and dermatologists to have access to quality and commented images, in order to know the typical characteristics of this new confocal microscopy semiology for the main types of tumors affecting this anatomical area.

In its design, it is a work modelled on the classic great books of anatomopathology that show the characteristic aspects of the different types of lesions.

Confocal microscopy has a reputation of expensive technique requiring a difficult training and thus reserved for a few experts. We hope that this book will demonstrate, on one hand, that the images are not difficult to be interpreted and, on the other hand, that the system can be shared by two disciplines in order to pool the costs. In vivo confocal microscopy offers the clinician an additional help for the diagnostic and therapeutic management of the anterior ocular tumors, thus avoiding unnecessary excisions of benign lesions such as conjunctival naevi and supporting the clinical diagnosis of malignant tumors.

In conclusion, although current devices provide high-quality images at cellular resolution, we hope that the confocal microscopy and optics industries will be able to continue to develop new devices that are more efficient and less expensive than those currently available to us. We also hope that a future book will be published in a few years, as a result of international collaborations within a network of "confocalists" specialized in lesions of the anterior ocular system.

We cannot conclude this preface without mentioning that this book is the result of the collaboration between dermatology and ophthalmology, two disciplines that are closely linked by confocal microscopy, and it is also the testimony of a deep friendship that enabled us to acquire a common medical culture that we wish to share with our readers.

Loire, France Jean-Luc Perrot
Siena, Italy Elisa Cinotti

Contents

Part I

Prerequisites to Confocal Microscopy for the Human Eye

An Introduction to In Vivo Confocal Microscopy

1

Mathilde Kaspi, Thibaud Garcin, Bruno Labeille, Michele Fimiani, Jean-Luc Perrot, and Elisa Cinotti

Content

Abbreviations

3D	Three dimensions
IVCM	In vivo reflectance confocal microscopy

Confocal microscopy was first described by the American scientist Marvin Minsky and patented in 1955.

In confocal microscopy, the detection and illumination systems are focused in the same focal plane. The light reflected by the elements outside the focal plane is eliminated; thus, images of high resolution (in the micron range) but of very limited depth (<500 μm) are obtained [1].

The simplified operating principles of the reflectance confocal microscope are as follows (Fig. 1.1) [2]:

- *Step 1*: An infrared laser excitation light source (830 nm for the Vivascope 3000® confocal microscope, by Caliber) is emitted and reflected by a dichroic mirror to be directed toward the galvanometric scanning mirrors. The dichroic mirror is an interference mirror that reflects certain wavelengths of a light beam and transmits other wavelengths. The scanning mirrors rotate on their axis to allow complete scanning of the focal plane to be studied (on the *x*- and *y*-axes).
- *Step 2*: The excitation light source passes through the capacitor (which is integrated into the microscope objective). The capacitor consists of a pinhole focusing the light source on a small point on the focal plane of the area under examination.
- *Step 3*: The emission light corresponds to the reflection of the laser beam by the elements of the sample under examination. Some of the reflected emission light passes through the lens (which is also integrated into the microscope objective) and is focused on

M. Kaspi (✉) · T. Garcin
Department of Ophthalmology, University Hospital of Saint-Etienne, Saint-Etienne Cedex 2, France
e-mail: mathilde.kaspi@gmail.com; garcinthibaud@gmail.com

B. Labeille · J.-L. Perrot
Department of Dermatology, University Hospital of Saint-Etienne, Saint-Etienne Cedex 2, France
e-mail: bruno.labeille@chu-st-etienne.fr; j.luc.perrot@chu-st-etienne.fr

M. Fimiani · E. Cinotti
Department of Dermatology, University of Siena, S. Maria alle Scotte Hospital, Siena, Italy
e-mail: michele.fimiani@unisi.it; elisa.cinotti@unisi.it

© Springer Nature Switzerland AG 2020
M. Kaspi et al. (eds.), *Eyelid and Conjunctival Tumors*,
https://doi.org/10.1007/978-3-030-36606-3_1

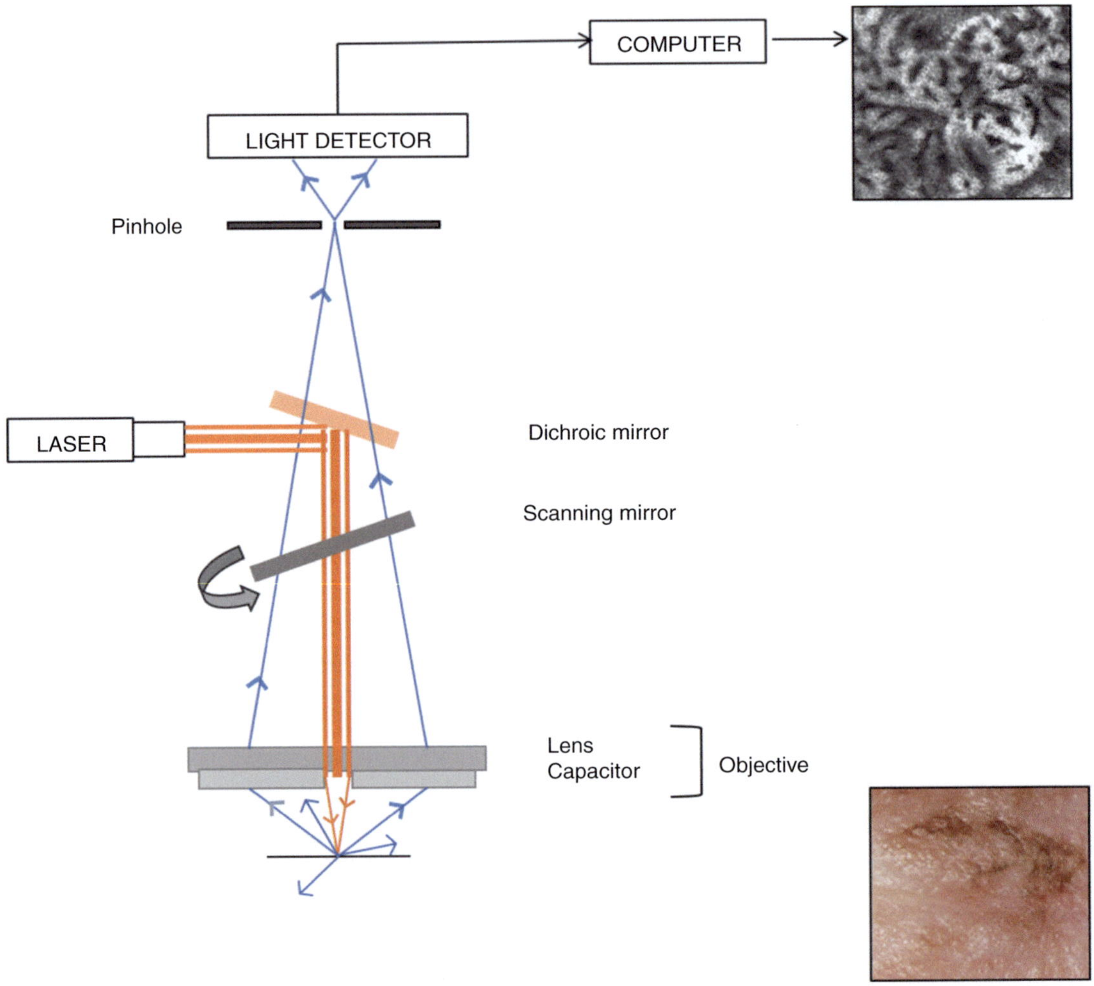

Fig. 1.1 Simplified operating principle of reflectance confocal microscopy

another focus in front of the light detector. The emission light also passes through the dichroic mirror, which, because of its function, separates the emission light and the reflected excitation light. The excitation light is reflected back to the sample under examination, while the emission light is transmitted to the light detector. The emission light passes through a pinhole before reaching the light detector.

- *Step 4*: Each analyzed element emits its own reflectance. The light detector separates these reflectances and associates a grayscale with them, thus giving a two-dimensional grayscale optical section (x- and y-axes). By moving the focal plane in the depth (z-axis), optical sections at different depths are obtained. These stacks of images can be analyzed by software and reconstructed in three dimensions (3D) (the unit image is then the voxel).

The in vivo reflectance confocal microscope used to produce the images in this book is a Vivascope 3000® V2 (Caliber, USA; distributed in Europe by Mavig, Germany). This microscope is equipped with a fixed camera and a manual camera. The latter is mobile and can be directly applied by an experienced operator to any area of the human body. It is usually dedicated to superficial examination of the skin and mucous membranes—in particular, by natural reflection of melanin [2, 3]. This reflectance confocal microscope has been developed for dermatology and allows exploration of the epidermis and papillary dermis up to 200–300 μm deep, with high resolution at the cellular scale, in the order of 1 μm [1, 2], close to that obtained by an optical microscope on histological sections [1].

In vivo reflectance confocal microscopy (IVCM) provides grayscale optical sections of the structure passed through, in vivo and in real time. It can be likened to virtual biopsy. The semiology of IVCM is based on that of histopathology [1]. Good anatomopathological knowledge is therefore essential for the interpretation of IVCM images.

Optical properties: The studied surface remains restricted (885 × 885 μm for the Vivascope 3000®), and a scan of the entire lesion is necessary to examine it in its entirety. The resolution of the Vivascope 3000® is 1000 × 1000 pixels. The theoretical magnification is ×392.

Practically speaking, a tip protects the microscope objective of the Vivascope 3000®. At the University Hospital of Saint-Etienne in France, a resterilizable tip has been created, but this has not yet been marketed. In the absence of a resterilizable tip, it must be disinfected in accordance with the same procedures that are used in ophthalmology for disinfecting examination lenses in contact with the cornea (e.g., Goldmann three-mirror lenses). The camera is directly applied to the area to be imaged after local anesthesia of the ocular surface (Fig. 1.2) (e.g., by application of oxybuprocaine and tetracaine eye drops (Théa, Clermont-Ferrand, France)) and aqueous gel (e.g., Gel-larmes; Théa) [4].

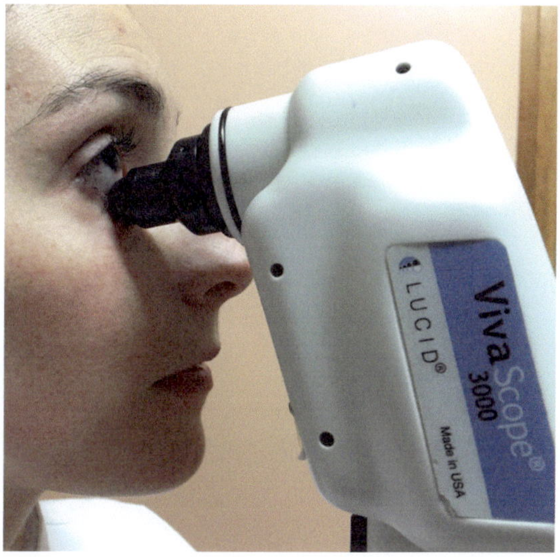

Fig. 1.2 In vivo reflectance confocal microscopy examination of the free edge of the eyelid

References

1. Kanitakis J, Bahadoran P, Braun R, Debarbieux S, Labeille B, Perrot J-L, et al. La microscopie confocale par réflectance in vivo en dermatologie : proposition de terminologie en langue française. Ann Dermatol Vénéréologie. 2013;140(11):678–86.
2. Nwaneshiudu A, Kuschal C, Sakamoto FH, Anderson RR, Schwarzenberger K, Young RC. Introduction to confocal microscopy. J Invest Dermatol. 2012;132(12):e3.
3. Xiang W, Peng J, Song X, Xu A, Zhang D, Liu J, et al. In vivo visualization of honeycomb pattern, cobblestone pattern, ringed pattern, and dermal papillae by confocal laser scanning microscopy. Skin Res Technol. 2016;22(1):32–9.
4. Cinotti E, Singer A, Labeille B, Grivet D, Rubegni P, Douchet C, et al. Handheld in vivo reflectance confocal microscopy for the diagnosis of eyelid margin and conjunctival tumors. JAMA Ophthalmol. 2017;135(8):845–51.

The Normal Eyelid

2

Thibaud Garcin, Elisa Cinotti, Cyril Habougit, Damien Grivet, Pietro Rubegni, and Jean-Luc Perrot

Abbreviation

IVCM In vivo reflectance confocal microscopy

Anatomically (Fig. 2.1), the eyelid is separated into the anterior and posterior lamella. The separation between these two lamellae is visible at the gray-line level between the eyelashes and the orifice of the excretory channels of the Meibomius glands.

T. Garcin (✉) · D. Grivet
Department of Ophthalmology, University Hospital of Saint-Etienne, Saint-Etienne Cedex 2, France
e-mail: garcinthibaud@gmail.com; damien.grivet@chu-st-etienne.fr

E. Cinotti · P. Rubegni
Department of Dermatology, University of Siena, S. Maria alle Scotte Hospital, Siena, Italy
e-mail: elisa.cinotti@unisi.it; pietro.rubegni@gmail.com

C. Habougit
Department of Pathology, University Hospital of Saint-Etienne, Saint-Etienne Cedex 2, France
e-mail: cyril.habougit@chu-st-etienne.fr

J.-L. Perrot
Department of Dermatology, University Hospital of Saint-Etienne, Saint-Etienne Cedex 2, France
e-mail: j.luc.perrot@chu-st-etienne.fr

© Springer Nature Switzerland AG 2020
M. Kaspi et al. (eds.), *Eyelid and Conjunctival Tumors*, https://doi.org/10.1007/978-3-030-36606-3_2

The anterior lamella includes:

- The skin (epidermis and dermis); the palpebral skin is the thinnest in the human body.
- The orbicularis oculi muscle.

The posterior lamella includes:

- The tarsus.
- The tarsal conjunctiva.

Figure 2.2 shows clinical aspects of a normal eyelid.

The epidermis is keratinized squamous epithelium consisting of four layers successively from the surface to the depth: the stratum corneum, the stratum granulosum, the stratum spinosum, and the stratum basale (the deepest layer).

The dermis is composed of papillary and reticular layers. It is the seat of the hair follicles, sebaceous glands (Meibomius and Zeis glands), and sweat glands (Moll glands).

The orbicular muscle is a skeletal striated muscle. Its marginal bundle at the free edge is called the Riolan muscle. It ensures palpebral closure.

The levator palpebrae muscle of the upper eyelid and the *lower lid retractor muscle* of the lower eyelid ensure palpebral opening.

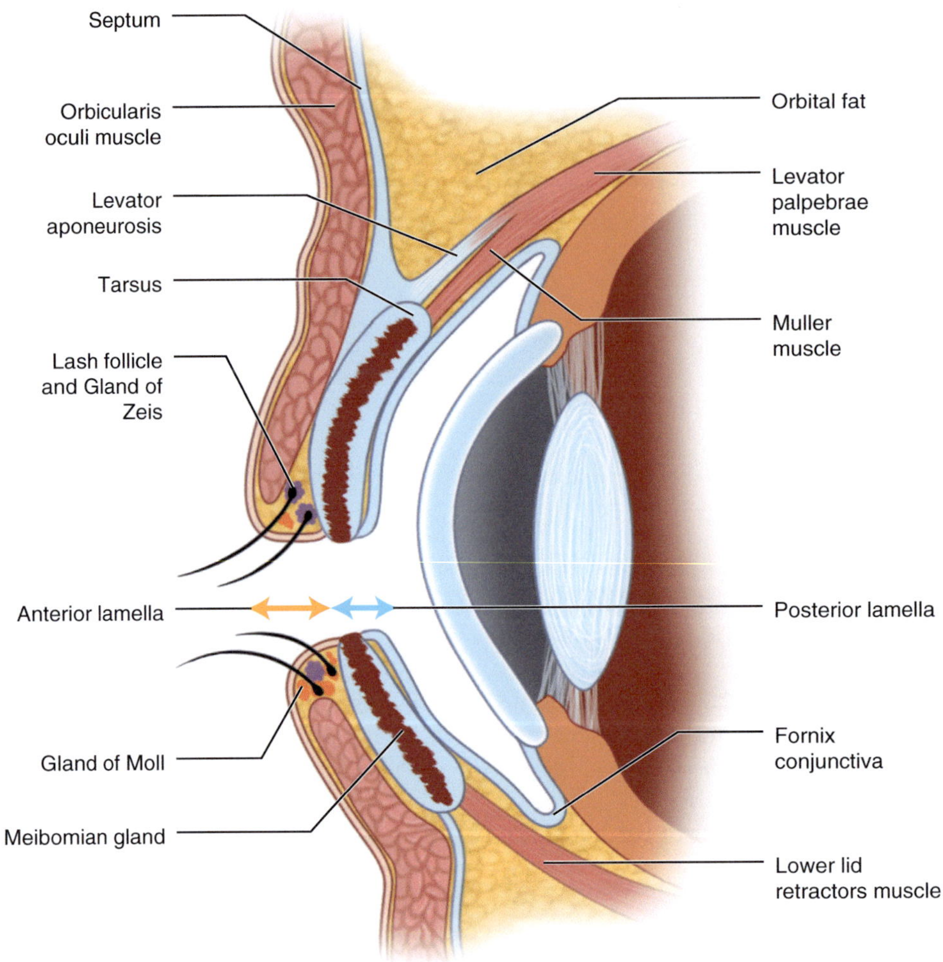

Fig. 2.1 Anatomical scheme of the eyelid

The Muller muscle is a smooth muscle going from the tendon of the levator palpebrae muscle to the tarsus. Its contraction allows the upper eyelid to be raised only by a few millimeters.

The septum is a thin fibrous blade that connects the orbital rim to the peripheral edge of the tarsus.

The tarsus consists of dense fibroelastic connective tissue. It is responsible for the stiffness of the eyelid.

The tarsal conjunctiva is composed of nonkeratinized laminated cylindrical epithelium with goblet cells that secrete the mucin component of the tear film.

The main glands are the Meibomius glands, the Zeis glands, and the Moll glands.

The Meibomius glands are sebaceous glands composed of several cells with an excretory channel ending at the free edge of the eyelids. They are

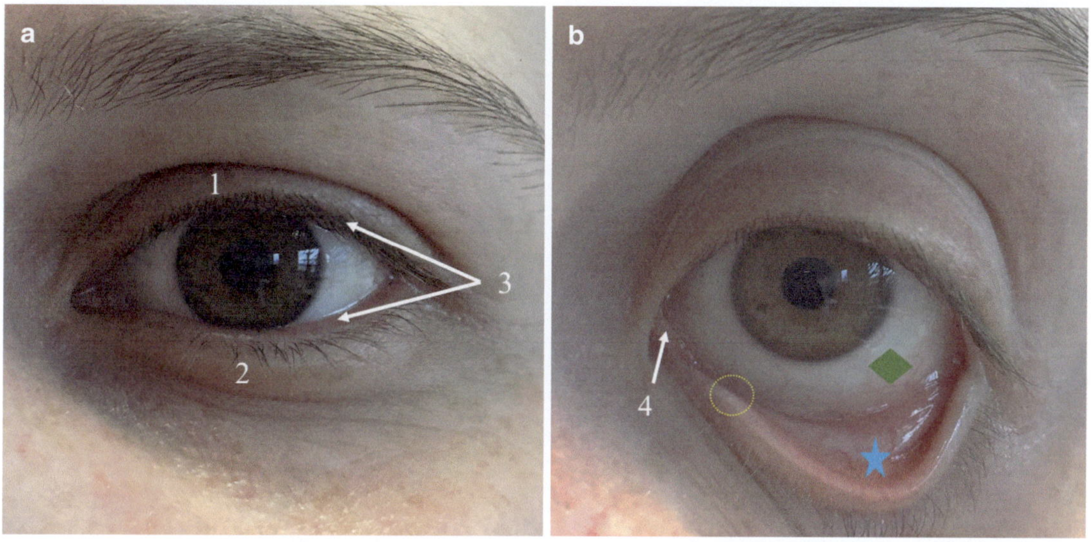

Fig. 2.2 (**a**) Normal eyelids viewed from the front: upper eyelid (*1*), lower eyelid (*2*), and free edges of the eyelids (*3*). (**b**) Normal reverse of lower eyelid: caruncle (*4*), lower tear puncta (*yellow circle*), bulbar conjunctiva (*green diamond*), and tarsal conjunctiva (*blue star*)

located in the tarsus. There are about 25 glands in the upper eyelid and 20 glands in the lower eyelid.

The Zeis glands are sebaceous glands in the infundibulum of the pilosebaceous follicle. The orifice of their excretory channel is common to that of the eyelash.

The Moll glands are apocrine sweat glands located between the pilosebaceous follicles.

Other examples include the accessory conjunctival tear glands (Krause and Wolfring glands), located between the tarsus and the fornix conjunctiva, which ensure basal aqueous lacrimal secretion.

Figure 2.3 shows features of a normal eyelid that are visible on in vivo reflectance confocal microscopy (IVCM). The IVCM features are as follows (Fig. 2.3c–n): Skin side: The cutaneous epidermis is of a regular honeycomb architecture (*red stars*). The free edge (*yellow arrow*) is hyperreflective because of the presence of keratinocytes of the stratum corneum and skin debris (*dashed green oval*). The eyelash shaft (*pale blue arrow*) is highly hyperreflective. The dermoepidermal junction (*orange diamonds*) is composed of rings delimiting a discreetly hyporeflective zone corresponding to the tip of dermal papillae in the areas with epithelial rete ridges (mainly on the cutaneous side), whereas this is not visible in the areas with a flattened epithelium (mainly on the conjunctival side). (i–n) Tarsal side: The tarsal conjunctival epithelium has a regular honeycomb architecture (*red stars*). The conjunctival chorion is characterized by the presence of regular thin and elongated hyperreflective fibers with a combed appearance (*pale blue crosses*). The lumen of the lower tear duct is hyporeflective (*yellow oval*). A Meibomian gland opening is visible (*pale orange arrows*).

Figure 2.4 shows histological features of a normal eyelid that are visible on optical microscopy. On optical microscopy the histologic features are as follows (Fig. 2.4o–v): cutaneous side (*I*), free edge (*II*), conjunctival side (*III*), orbicularis oculi muscle (*1*), epidermis (*2*) (composed of the stratum corneum (*a*), stratum granulosum (*b*), stratum spinosum (*c*), and stratum basale (*d*)), Moll gland (*3*), dermis (*4*), hair follicle (*5*), Zeis gland (*6*), Riolan muscle (*7*), tarsus (*8*), Meibomius gland (*9*), conjunctival epithelium (*10*), and goblet cells of the conjunctival epithelium (*11*).

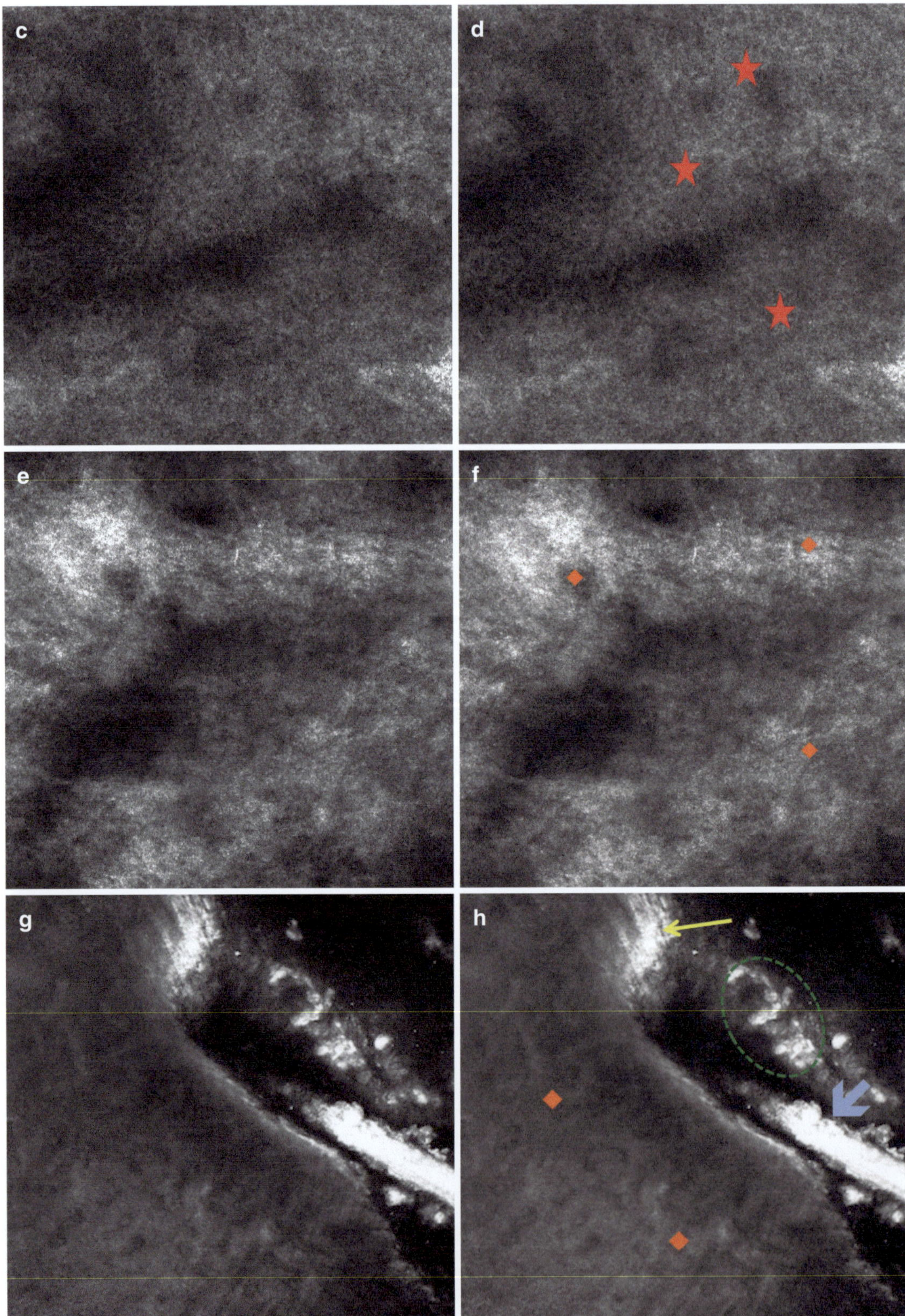

Fig. 2.3 In vivo reflectance confocal microscopy features of a normal eyelid

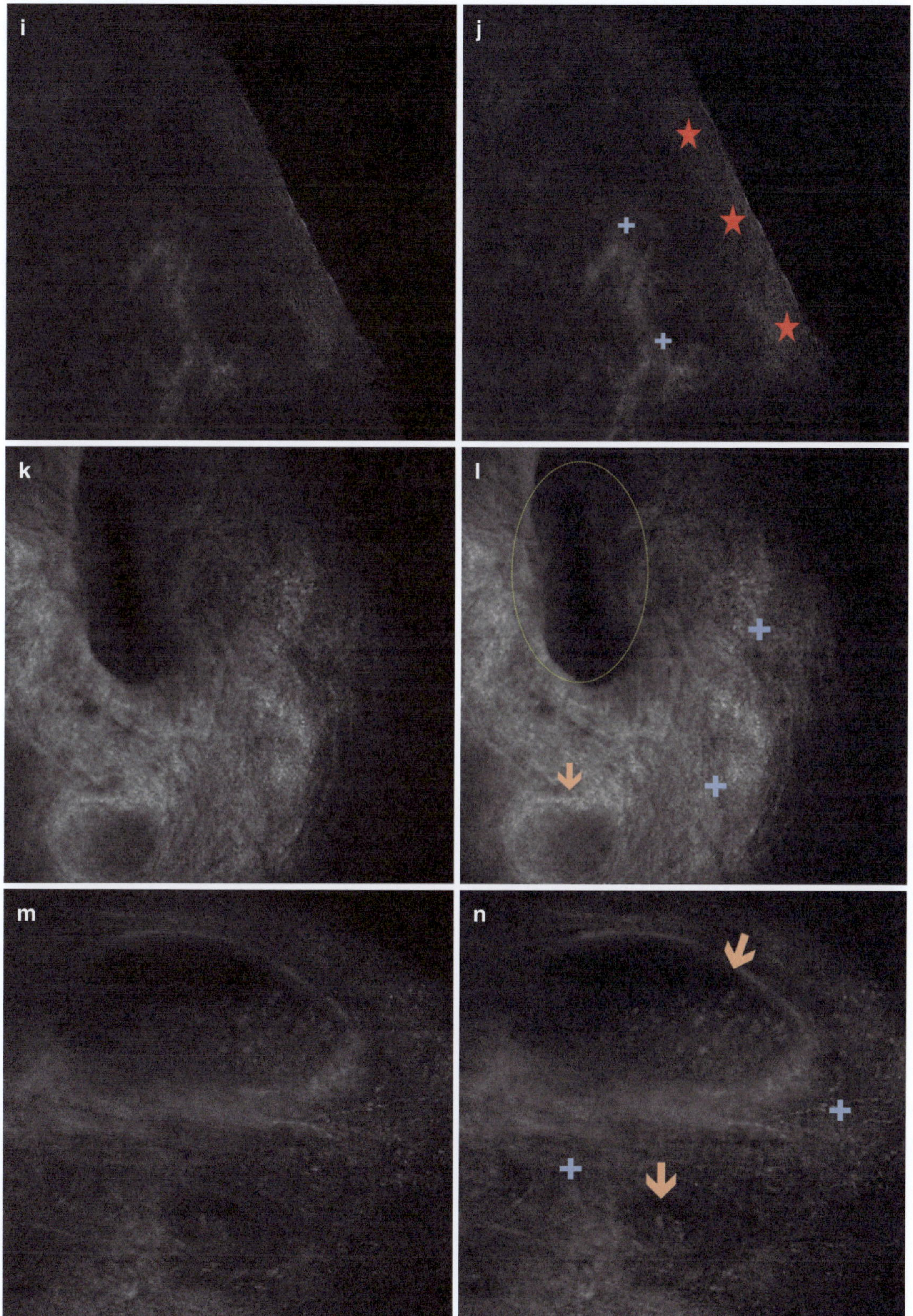

Fig. 2.3 (continued)

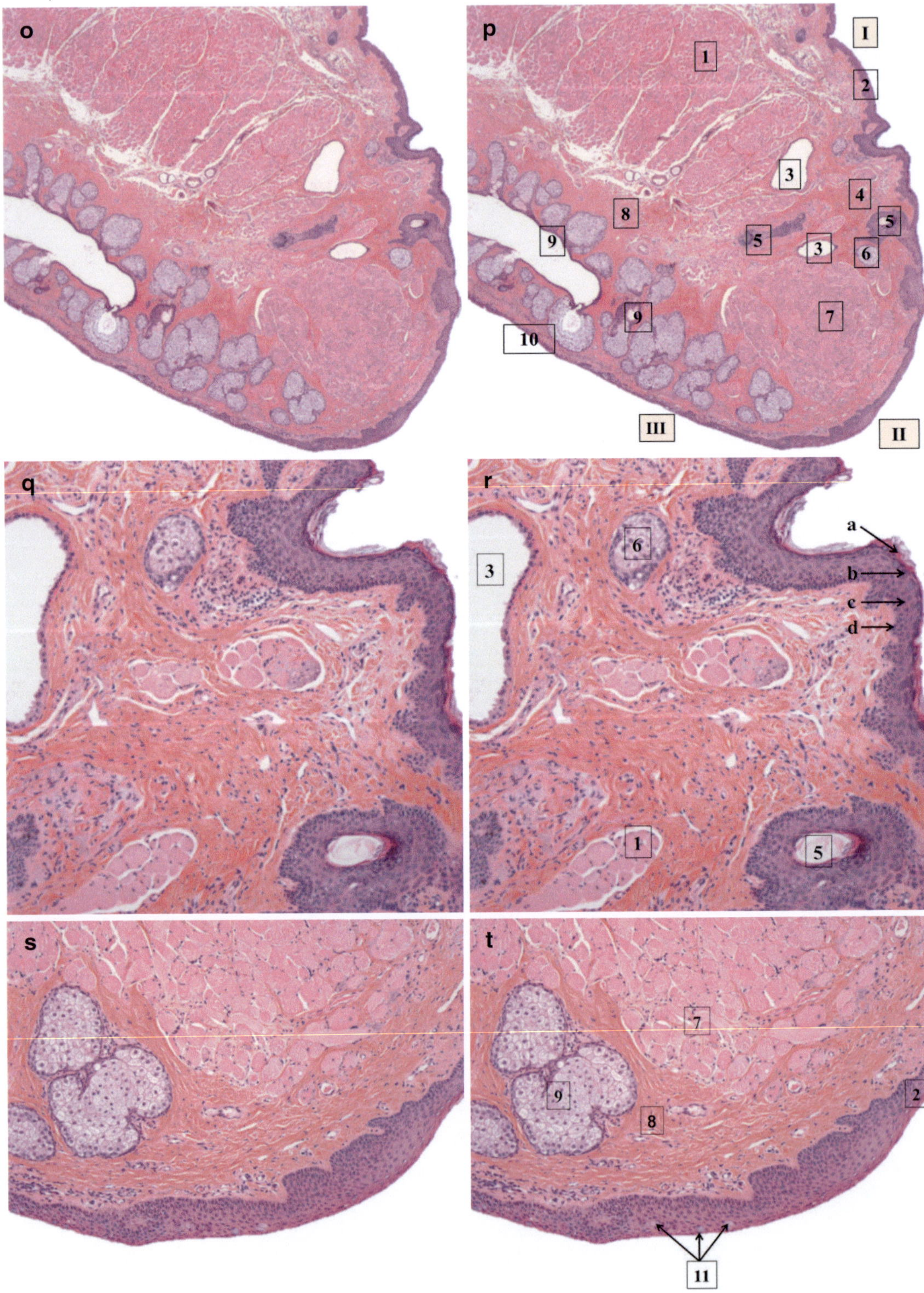

Fig. 2.4 Histological features of a normal eyelid, revealed with hematoxylin-eosin-saffron stain and magnifications

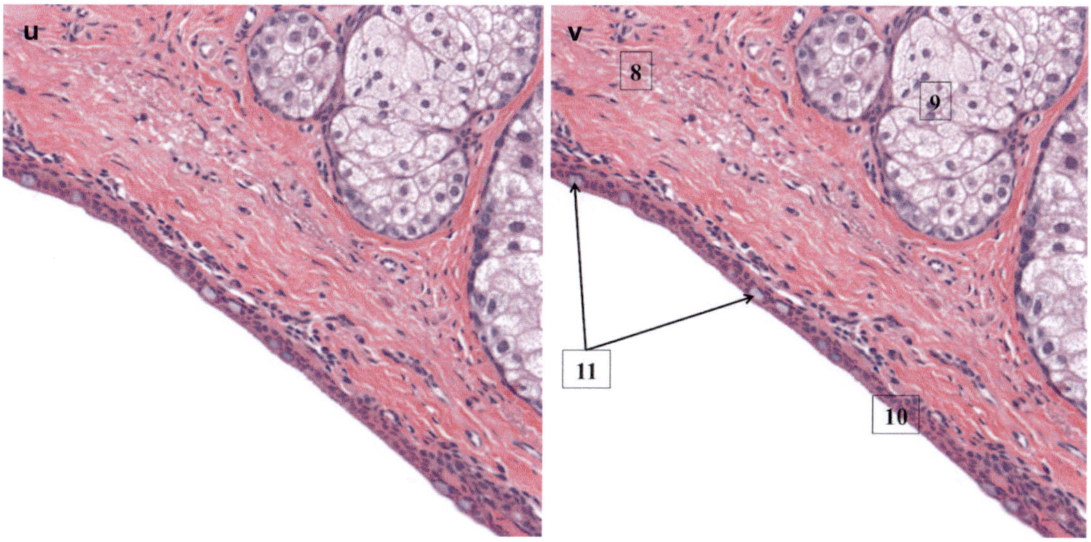

Fig. 2.4 (continued)

The Normal Conjunctiva

3

Thibaud Garcin, Mathilde Kaspi, Cyril Habougit, Elisa Cinotti, Michel Peoc'h, and Jean-Luc Perrot

Abbreviations

HES	Hematoxylin-eosin-saffron stain
IVCM	In vivo reflectance confocal microscopy

The conjunctiva is a mucous membrane or mucosa. It covers the sclera and tarsal face of the eyelids. The junction between the bulbar and tarsal conjunctiva forms the fornix conjunctiva (upper and lower).

The conjunctiva is composed of an epithelium and a substantia propria or chorion or stroma.

- The epithelium is nonkeratinized and stratified. It sits on a thin basal membrane. The specificity of the conjunctival epithelium is that it contains goblet cells, which secrete mucus. A normal epithelium contains some melanocytes, some Langerhans cells, and some lymphocytes.
- The chorion is composed of dense connective tissue and capillary, arterioles, and venules.

The conjunctiva is transparent and smooth and the two types are (Fig. 3.1) bulbar conjunctiva (*green diamond*) and tarsal conjunctiva (*blue star*).

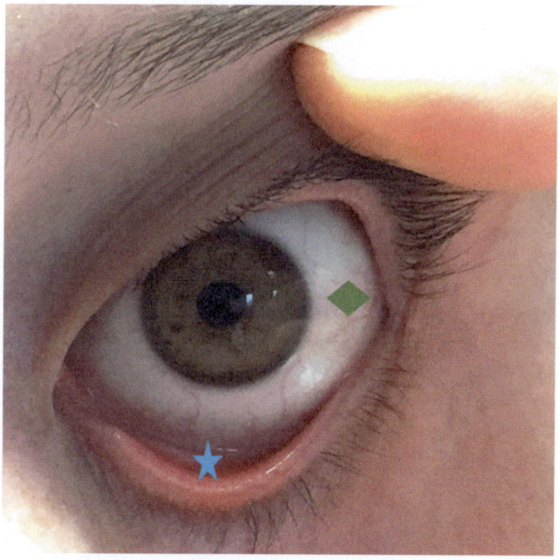

Fig. 3.1 Clinical aspect of normal conjunctiva

T. Garcin (✉) · M. Kaspi
Department of Ophthalmology, University Hospital of Saint-Etienne, Saint-Etienne Cedex 2, France
e-mail: garcinthibaud@gmail.com; mathilde.kaspi@gmail.com

C. Habougit · M. Peoc'h
Department of Pathology, University Hospital of Saint-Etienne, Saint-Etienne Cedex 2, France
e-mail: cyril.habougit@chu-st-etienne.fr; michel.peoc'h@chu-st-etienne.fr

E. Cinotti
Department of Dermatology, University of Siena, S. Maria alle Scotte Hospital, Siena, Italy
e-mail: elisa.cinotti@unisi.it

J.-L. Perrot
Department of Dermatology, University Hospital of Saint-Etienne, Saint-Etienne Cedex 2, France
e-mail: j.luc.perrot@chu-st-etienne.fr

© Springer Nature Switzerland AG 2020
M. Kaspi et al. (eds.), *Eyelid and Conjunctival Tumors*,
https://doi.org/10.1007/978-3-030-36606-3_3

The IVCM features are as follows (Fig. 3.2a–d):

- The epithelium (a) has a regular honeycomb architecture. The cells are polygonal, regular with a thin hyperreflective membrane, hyporeflective cytoplasm, and medium reflective round nuclei.
- In the underlying stroma (b, c), elongated hyperreflective structures are organized in a dense meshwork (corresponding to collagen fibers). Compared to the dermis of the skin, the collagen of the conjunctival stroma is denser and more reflective. Prominent capillaries are visible (*orange stars*).

Due to the convexity of the surface of the eye and a possible sliding of the conjunctiva on the sclera, some images show vertical sections with epithelium, epithelium-stroma junction, and stroma.

- Fluorescence (d) after injection of fluorescein contrast agent allows the conjunctival vascular tree to be identified.

On optical microscopy the histologic features are as follows (Fig. 3.3e–j):

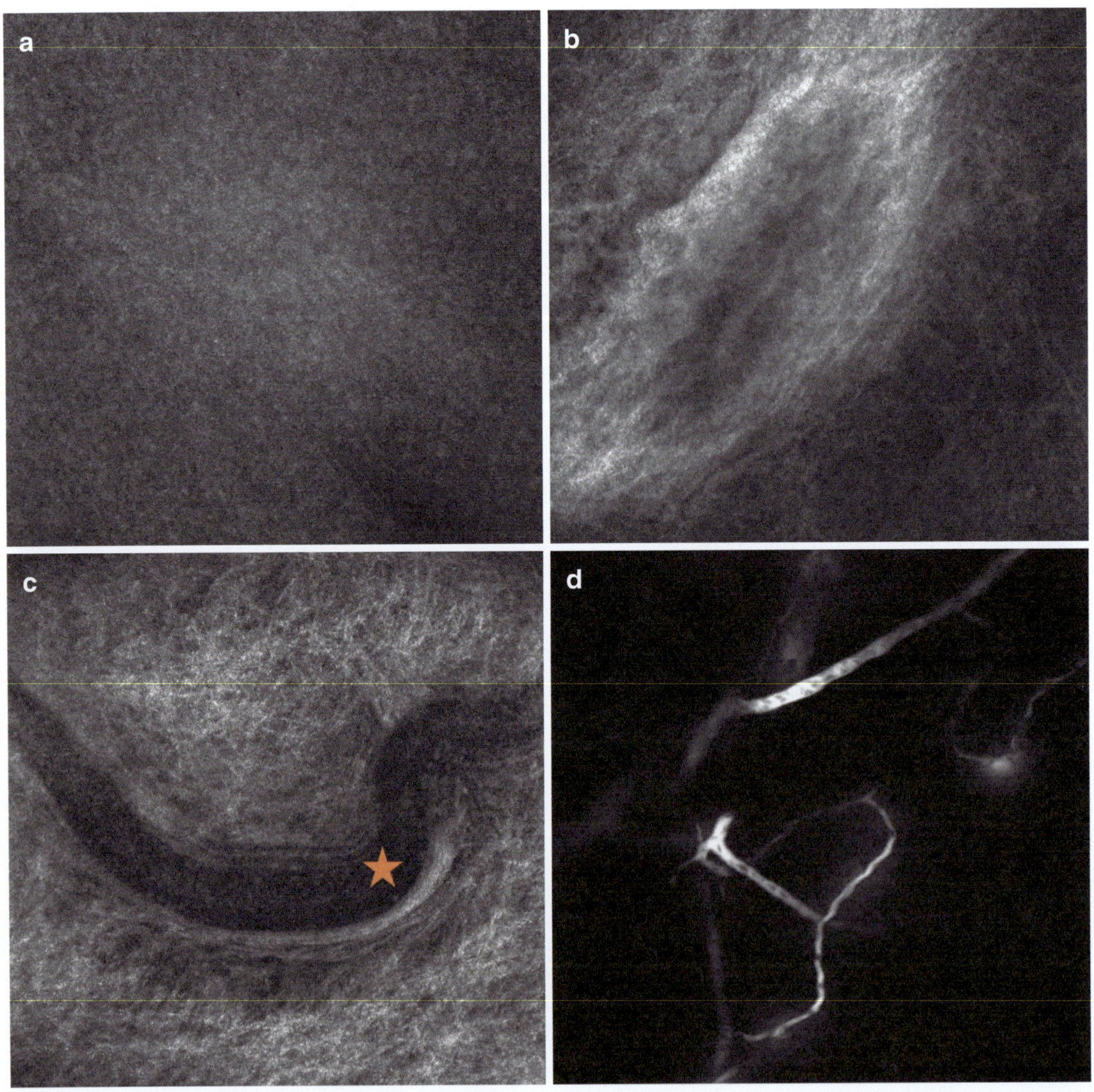

Fig. 3.2 IVCM features of normal conjunctiva (**a**–**d**)

- Nonkeratinized stratified epithelium (*red stars*) is composed of several layers (3–5) of cylindrical or cuboidal cells. The goblet cells (*black arrows*) are located within the epithelium. These cells appear large, round, and light in the HES staining and their cytoplasm is well identified by the Alcian Blue staining (i, j).
- Basal membrane (*dotted green*).
- Underlying chorion with dense connective tissue (*yellow diamonds*) and vessels (*orange stars*).

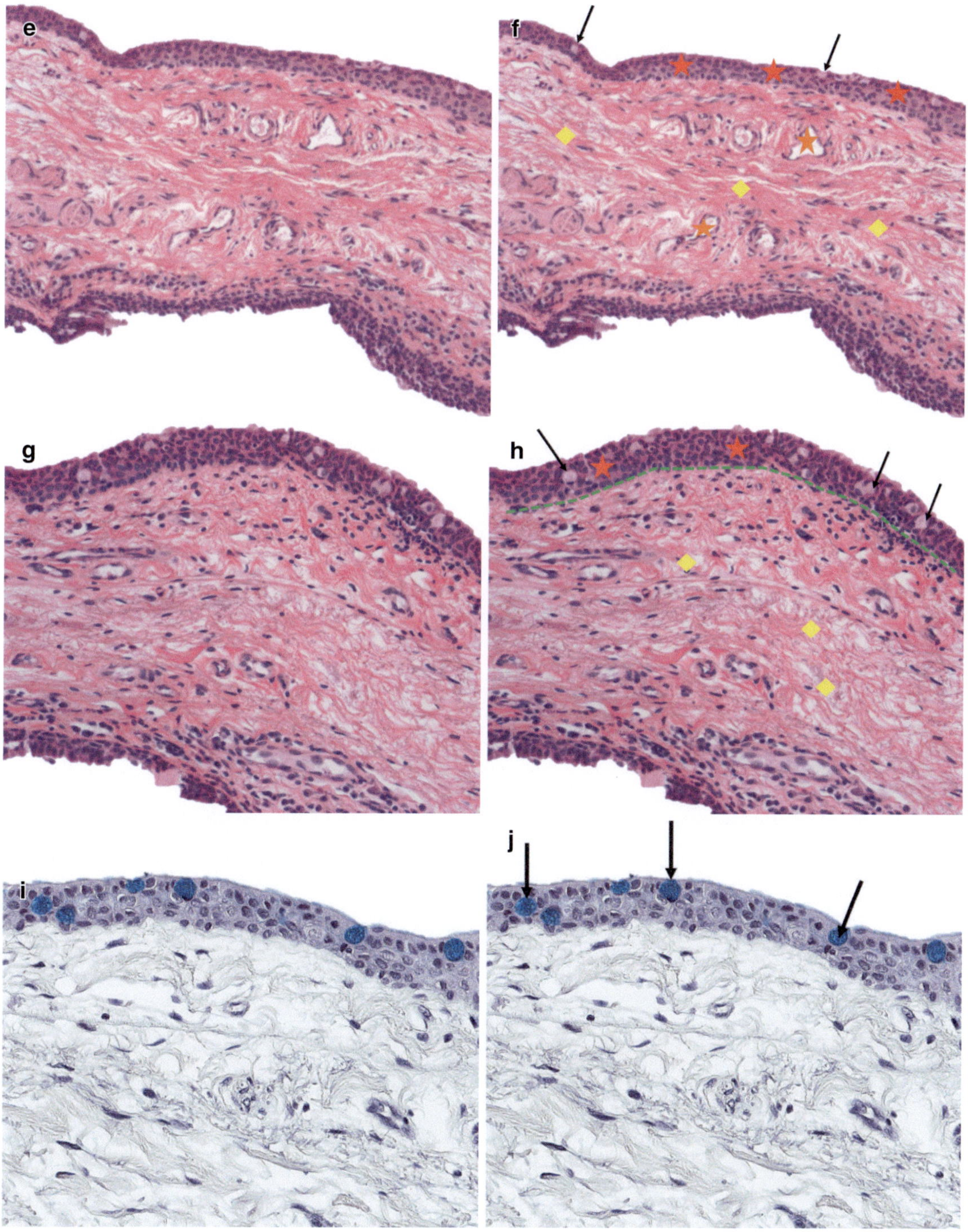

Fig. 3.3 Histological features of normal conjunctiva (**e–j**). (**e**, **f**) ×100 HES. (**g**, **h**) ×200 HES. (**i**, **j**) ×200 Alcian Blue staining

Part II

Epidermal Lesions of the Eyelid

Benign Epidermal Lesions

4

Mathilde Kaspi, Thibaud Garcin, Cyril Habougit, Damien Grivet, Elisa Cinotti, Fabien Forest, and Jean-Luc Perrot

Contents

Abbreviations

Ab	Antibodies
HES	Hematoxylin-eosin-saffron stain
IVCM	In vivo reflectance confocal microscopy

M. Kaspi (✉) · T. Garcin · D. Grivet
Department of Ophthalmology, University Hospital of Saint-Etienne, Saint-Etienne Cedex 2, France
e-mail: mathilde.kaspi@gmail.com; garcinthibaud@gmail.com; damien.grivet@chu-st-etienne.fr

C. Habougit · F. Forest
Department of Pathology, University Hospital of Saint-Etienne, Saint-Etienne Cedex 2, France
e-mail: cyril.habougit@chu-st-etienne.fr; fabien.forest@chu-st-etienne.fr

E. Cinotti
Department of Dermatology, University of Siena, S. Maria alle Scotte Hospital, Siena, Italy
e-mail: elisa.cinotti@unisi.it

J.-L. Perrot
Department of Dermatology, University Hospital of Saint-Etienne, Saint-Etienne Cedex 2, France
e-mail: j.luc.perrot@chu-st-etienne.fr

© Springer Nature Switzerland AG 2020
M. Kaspi et al. (eds.), *Eyelid and Conjunctival Tumors*,
https://doi.org/10.1007/978-3-030-36606-3_4

4.1 Papilloma

The clinical aspect (Fig. 4.1) of the papilloma is exophytic, pedunculated, or sessile. Papilloma can be single or multiple. It is most often flesh colored but it can be pigmented.

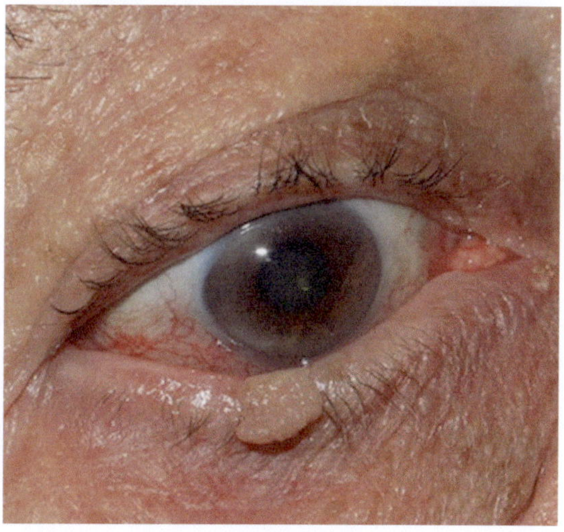

Fig. 4.1 Clinical aspect of papilloma

The IVCM features are as follows (Fig. 4.2a–d):

- Papillomatous epidermis (*yellow dotted lines*) with regular honeycomb pattern (*red stars*) (a, b)
- Dermo-epidermal junction (c, d) in the form of stretched rings or polycyclic papillary contours bordered by bright cells (*orange arrows*)

On optical microscopy the histologic features are as follows (Fig. 4.3e–h):

- At low magnification (e, f), papilloma shows a fibrovascular axis covered with pluristratified keratinized epithelium; the epidermis has a papillomatous architecture and its stratum corneum exhibits parakeratosis and hyperkeratosis (*green stars*).
- At high magnification (g, h), the epidermis is focally acanthotic (*black arrows*).

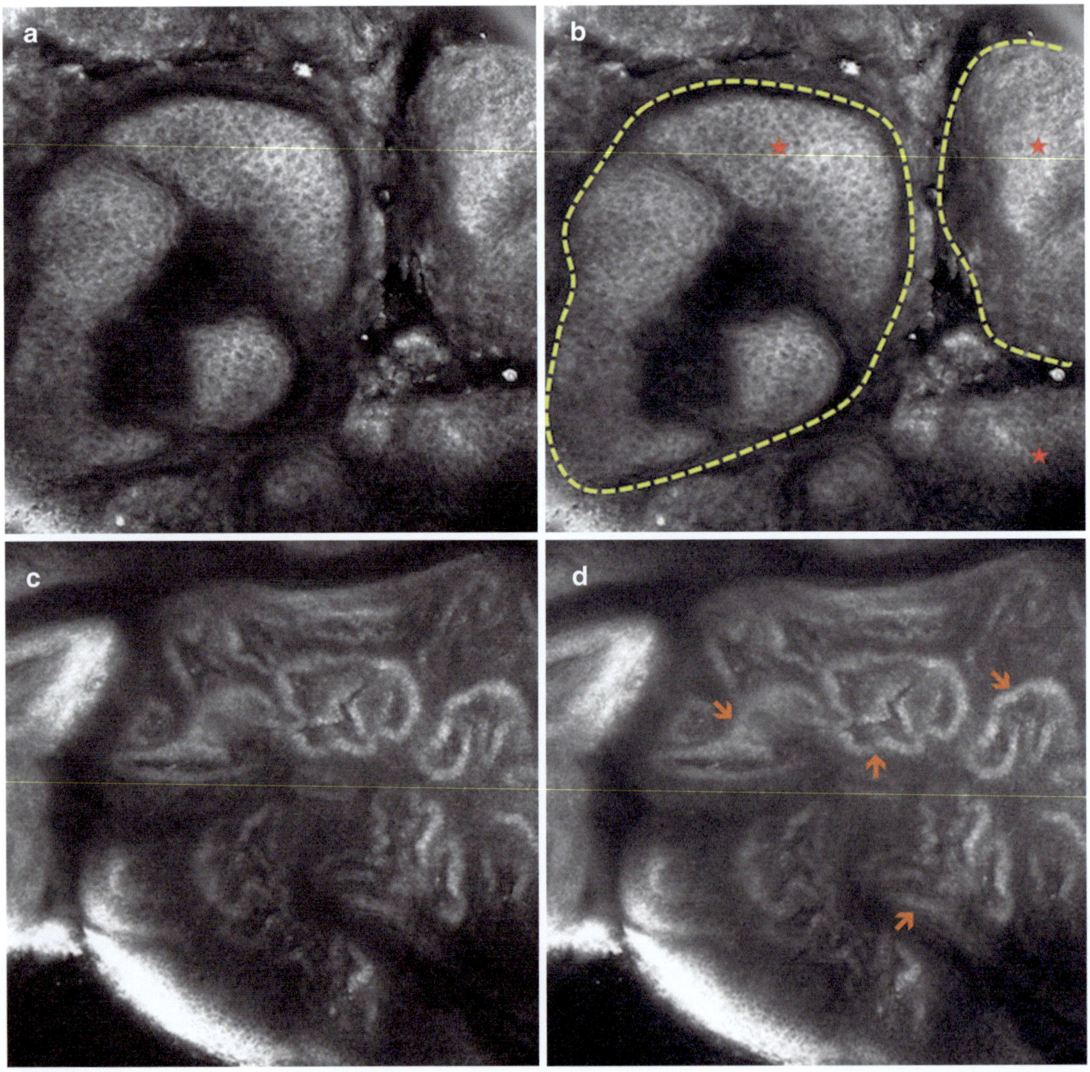

Fig. 4.2 IVCM features of papilloma (**a–d**)

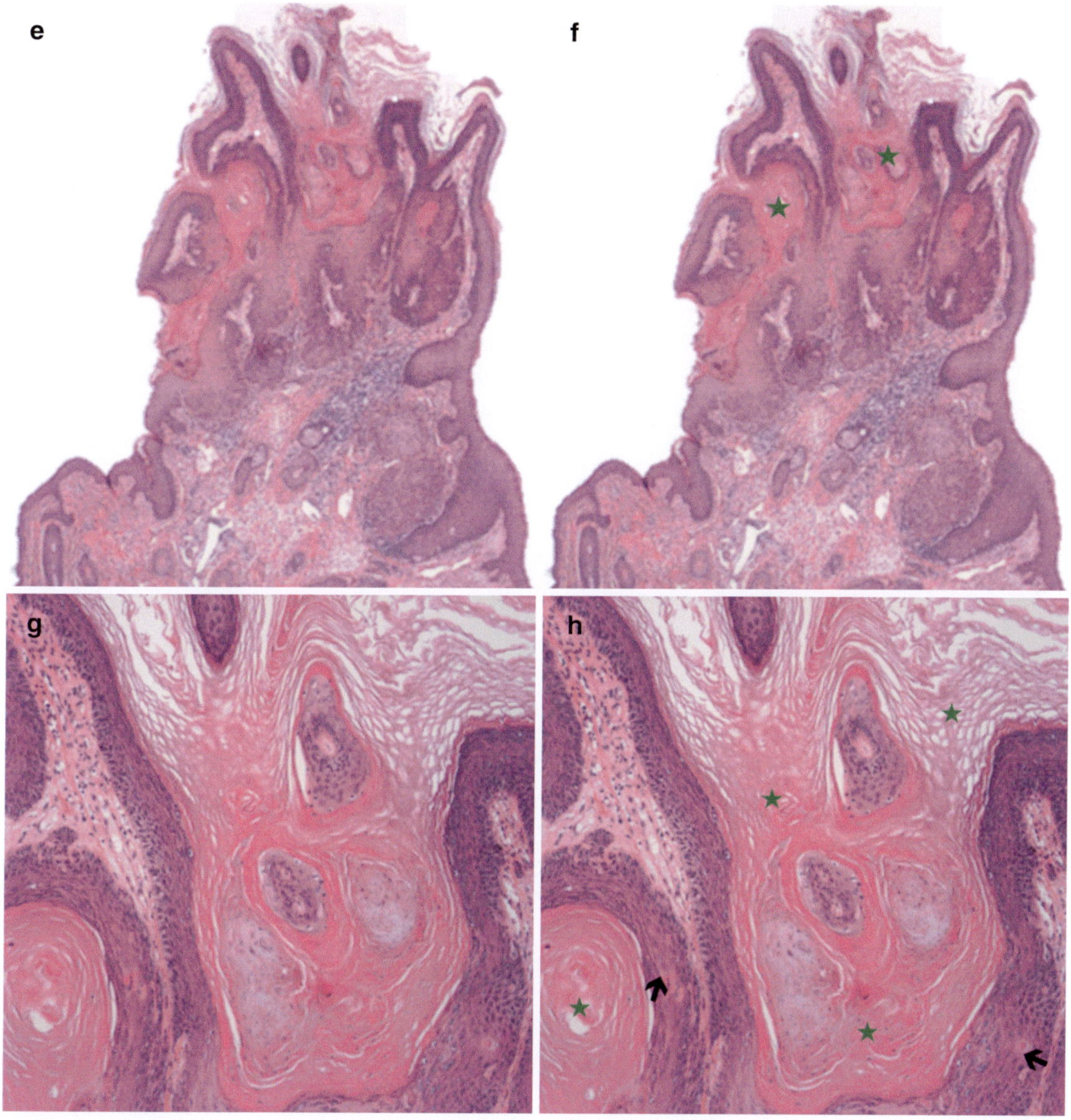

Fig. 4.3 Histological features of papilloma (**e**–**h**). (**e**, **f**) ×25 HES. (**g**, **h**) ×100 HES

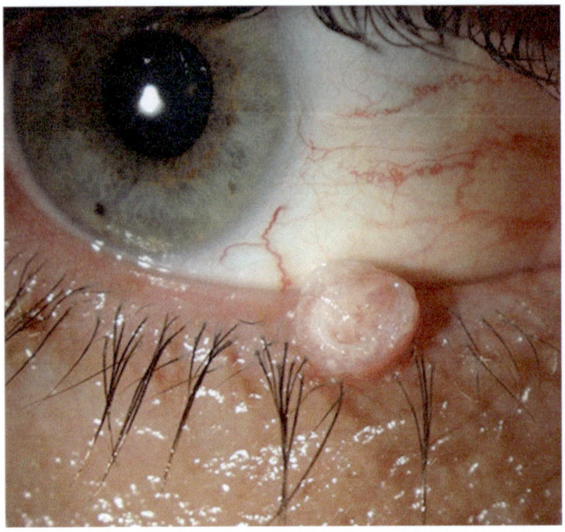

Fig. 4.4 Clinical aspect of wart: slit-lamp photography

4.2 Wart

Wart (Fig. 4.4) usually appears as a delineated papule or nodule, covered by keratotic surface. Its color is whitish or pinkish and more rarely pigmented. Its origin is viral due to Human Papilloma Virus infection.

The IVCM features are as follows (Fig. 4.5a–d):

- Papillomatous epidermis (*yellow dotted lines*) with irregular honeycomb pattern (*red stars*) with scattered large keratinocytes
- Hyperkeratosis of the stratum corneum of the epidermis (*blue arrows*)

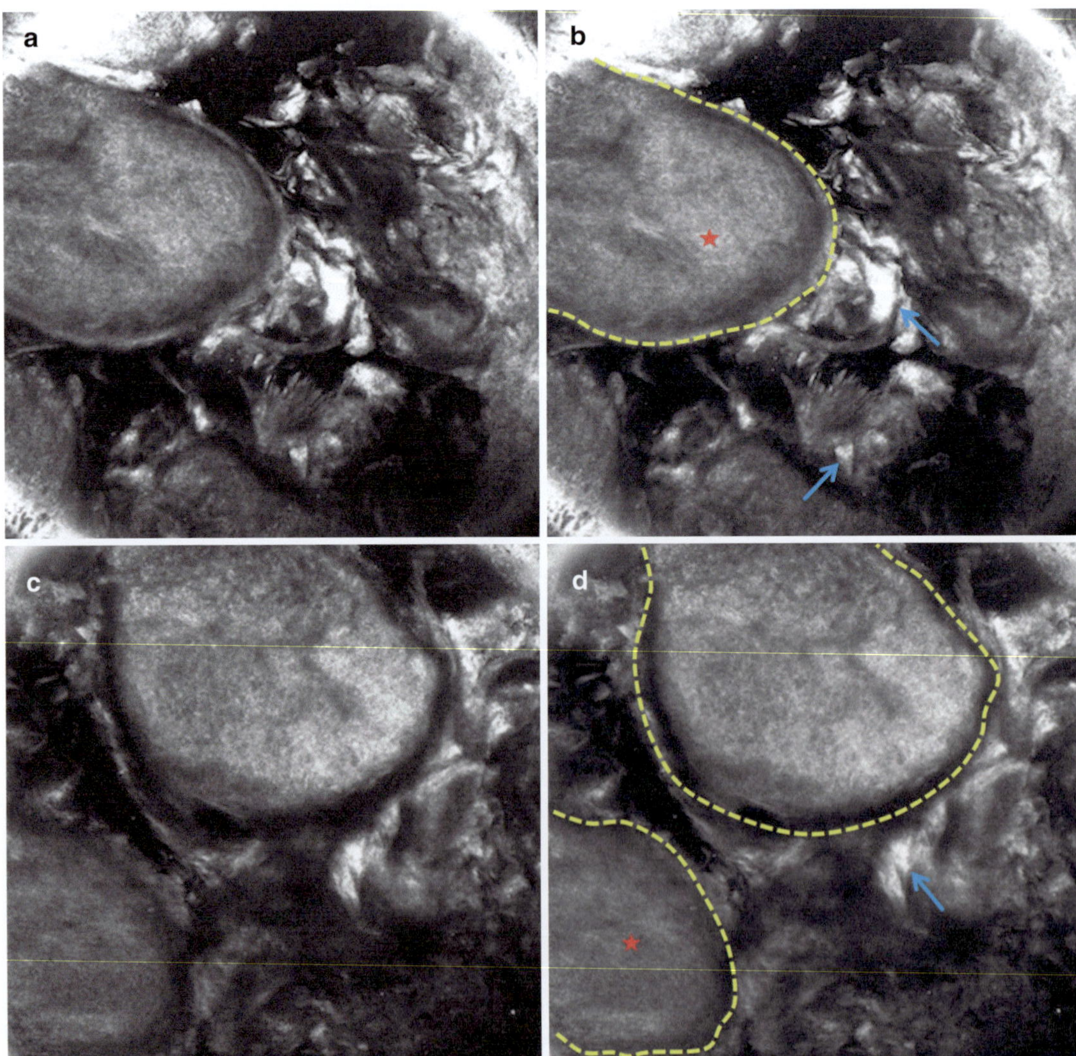

Fig. 4.5 IVCM features of wart (**a**–**d**)

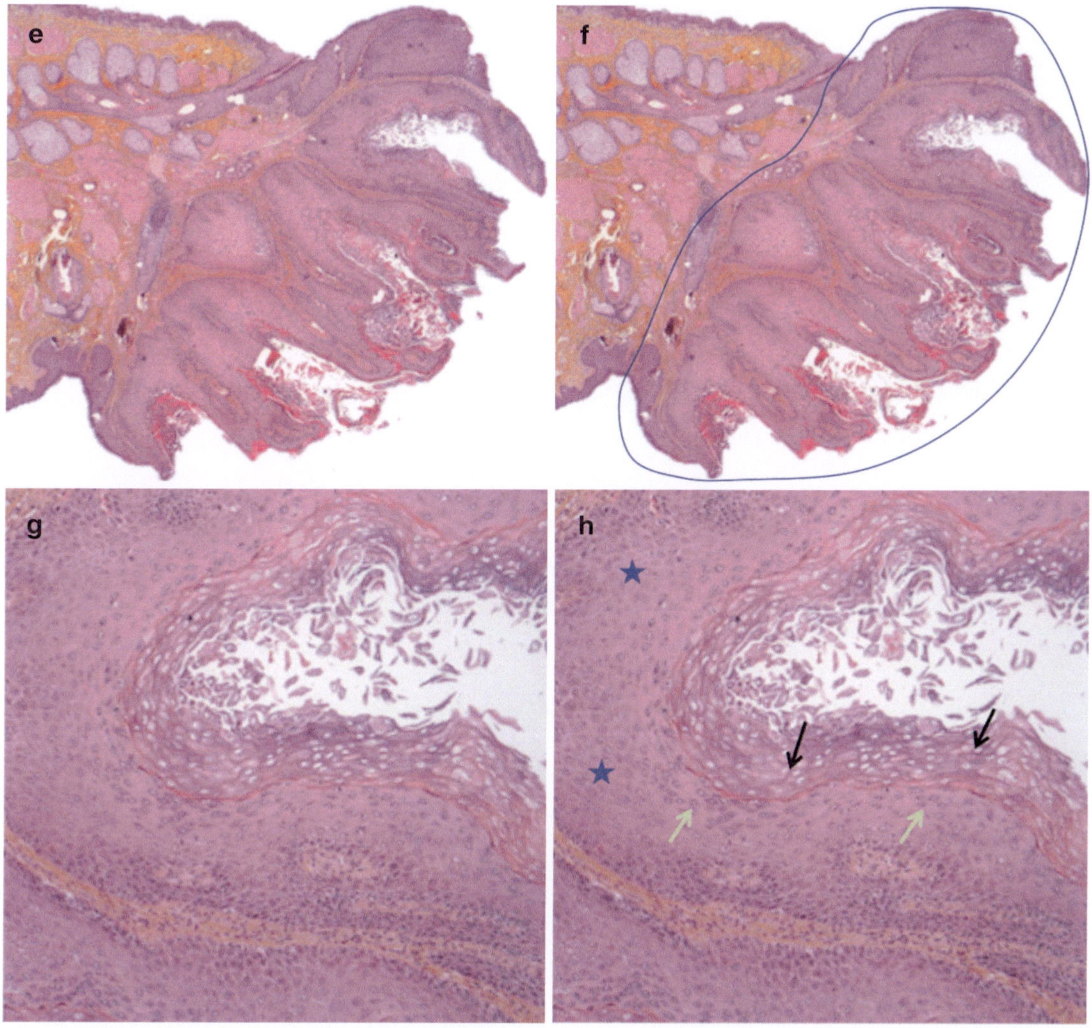

Fig. 4.6 Histological features of wart (**e**–**h**). (**e**, **f**) ×25 HES. (**g**, **h**) ×100 HES

On optical microscopy the histologic features are as follows (Fig. 4.6e–h):

- At low magnification (e, f), an exophytic lesion with a clear lower limit covered by hyperkeratosis is seen (*blue line*).
- At high magnification (g, h), hyperkeratosis with keratohyaline granules (*black arrows*) is seen. The acanthotic, papillomatous epidermis contains an irregular granular layer (*blue stars*), as well as viral infection stigmas (superficial cells of the epidermis containing a large cytoplasm and viral inclusions) (*green arrows*).

4.3 Molluscum Contagiosum

The clinical aspect (Fig. 4.7) of molluscum contagiosum is a small translucent or dewy papule measuring a few millimeters in diameter. It has an umbilication in its center. Its origin is viral due to Pox virus. Recurrent episodes of conjunctivitis are frequently associated.

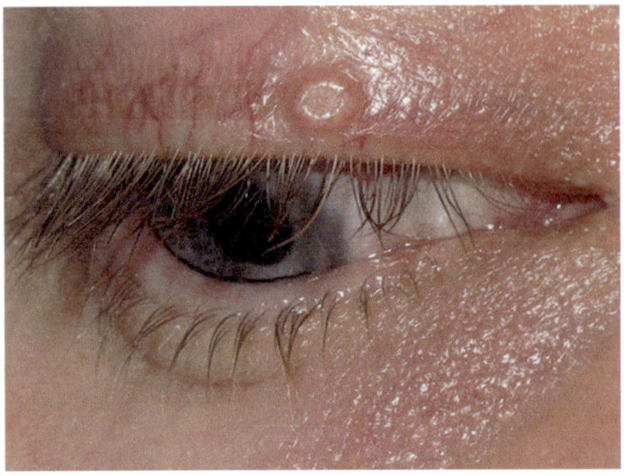

Fig. 4.7 Clinical aspect of molluscum contagiosum

The IVCM features are as follows (Fig. 4.8a–d):

- Round, well-circumscribed lesion with lobulated architecture.
- Pomegranate-like epidermis composed of multiple hyperreflective round cells (corresponding to molluscum bodies (*yellow stars*) separated by trabeculae.

On optical microscopy the histologic features are as follows (Fig. 4.9e–i):

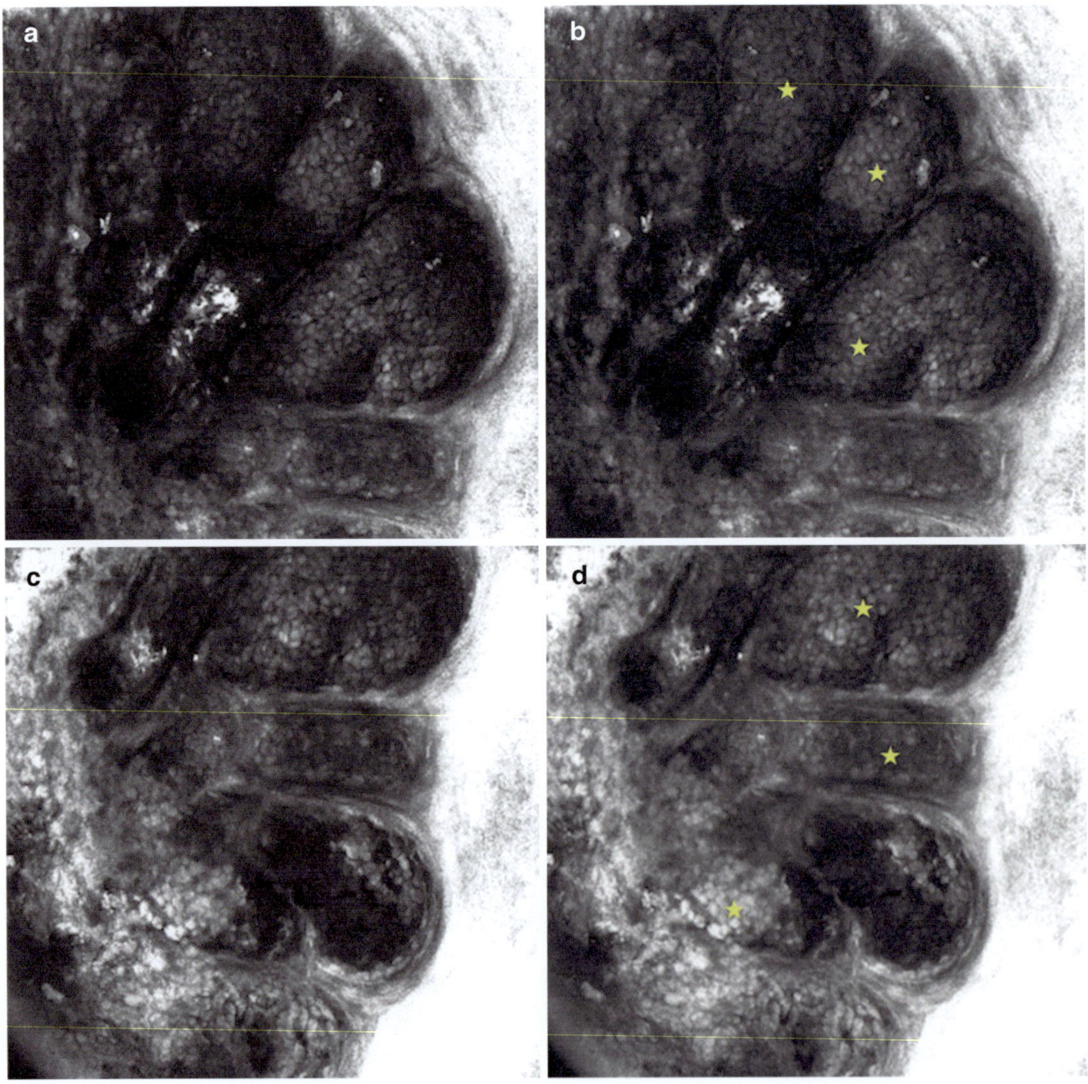

Fig. 4.8 IVCM features of molluscum contagiosum (**a–d**)

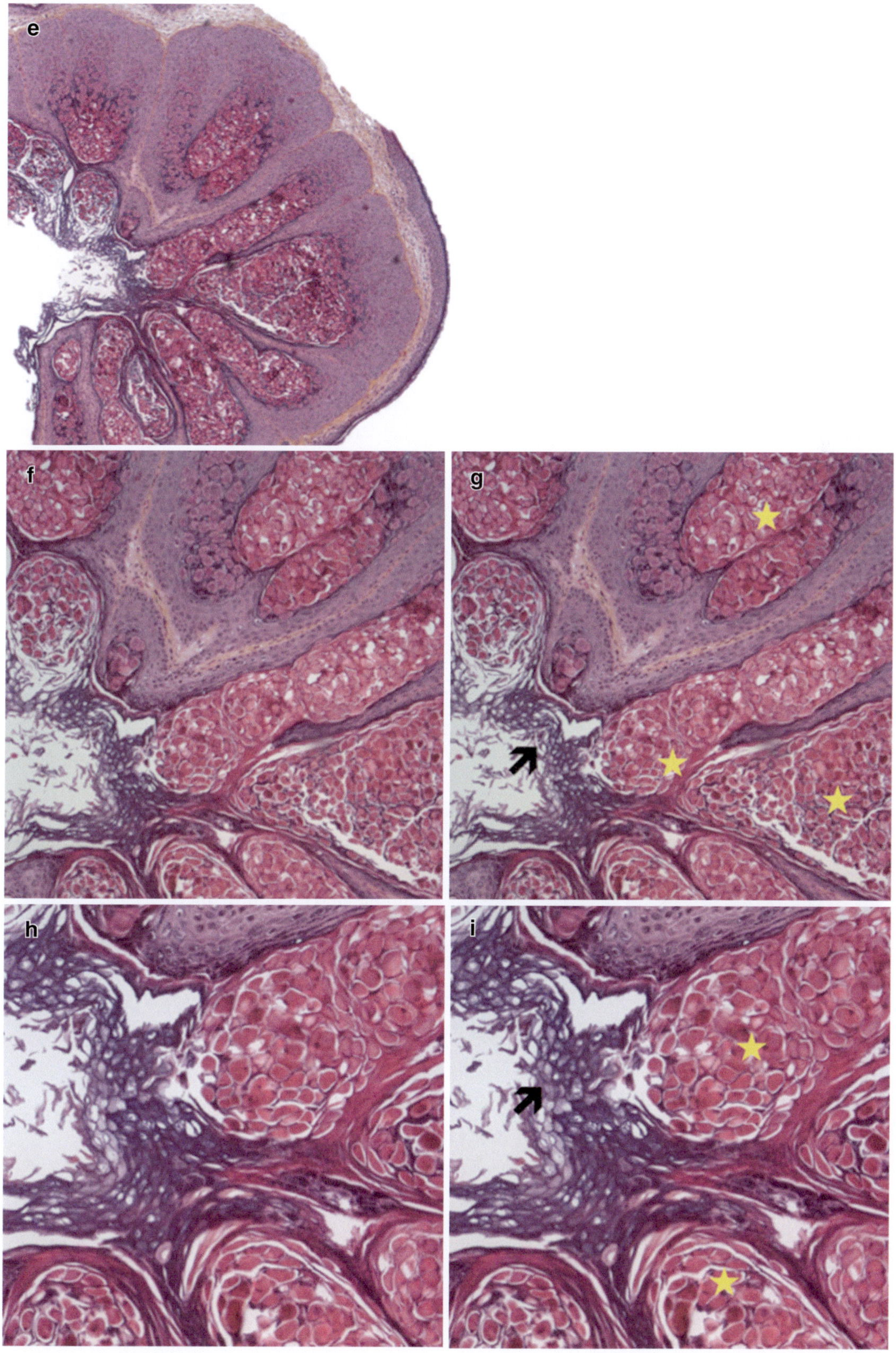

Fig. 4.9 Histological features of molluscum contagiosum (**e**–**i**). (**e**) ×50 HES. (**f**, **g**) ×100 HES. (**h**, **i**) ×200 HES

- At low magnification (e), epithelial hyperplasia is of lobulated architecture. The epidermal lobules invaginate in the dermis.
- At high magnification (f–i), the lobules contain infected keratinocytes presenting as hyaline corpuscles (Henderson-Patterson body or molluscum bodies (*yellow stars*)). Keratohyaline is pushed into the center of the lesion (*black arrows*).

4.4 Seborrheic Keratosis

The factors favoring seborrheic keratosis are genetic background, age, and sun exposure. It is a very common benign tumor. Its growth is slow.

The lesion is clinically well delineated, flat or raised, and sometimes pigmented.

Histologically, several forms are described:

- The acanthotic form (= common)
- The hyperkeratotic form (= papillomatous)
- The adenoid form (= reticulated)
- The clonal shape
- The irritated form with an inflammatory lichenoid reaction

We will illustrate the first three forms.

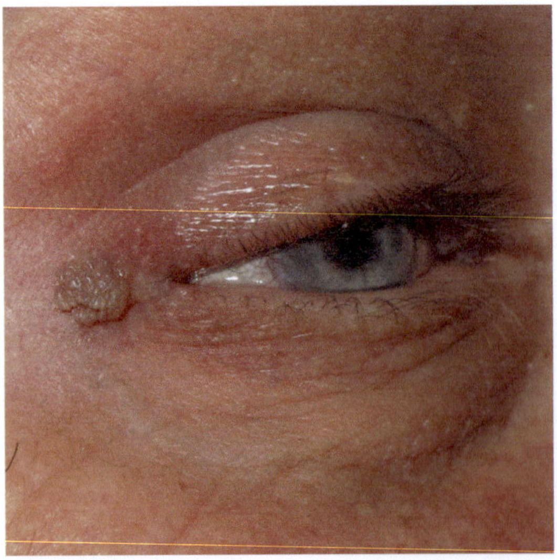

Fig. 4.10 Clinical aspect of common form of seborrheic keratosis

4.4.1 Seborrheic Keratosis: Common Form

The clinical aspect (Fig. 4.10) of a common form of seborrheic keratosis is a well-circumscribed pigmented or unpigmented papillomatous lesion.

The IVCM features are as follows (Fig. 4.11a–d):

- Widening and interweaving of the epidermal rete ridges (polycyclic papillary contours) (*yellow dotted lines*) while maintaining a regular honeycomb architecture (*red stars*)
- Horny pseudocysts in the epithelium
- Dermo-epidermal junction in the form of irregular rings (polycyclic papillary contours) bordered by small bright and regular keratinocytes (*orange arrows*)
- Superficial dermis consisting of normal and bright plump cells corresponding to melanophages

On optical microscopy the histologic features are as follows (Fig. 4.12e–h):

- At low magnification (e, f), an exophytic epidermal proliferation is seen, with a clear lower limit (*black dotted line*), a hyperplastic epithelium arranged in anastomotic cords containing islets of dermal conjunctiva (*blue stars*), and horny pseudocysts (*black arrows*).
- At high magnification (g, h), surface hyperkeratosis is minimal. Some epithelial cells are pigmented (*yellow arrows*).

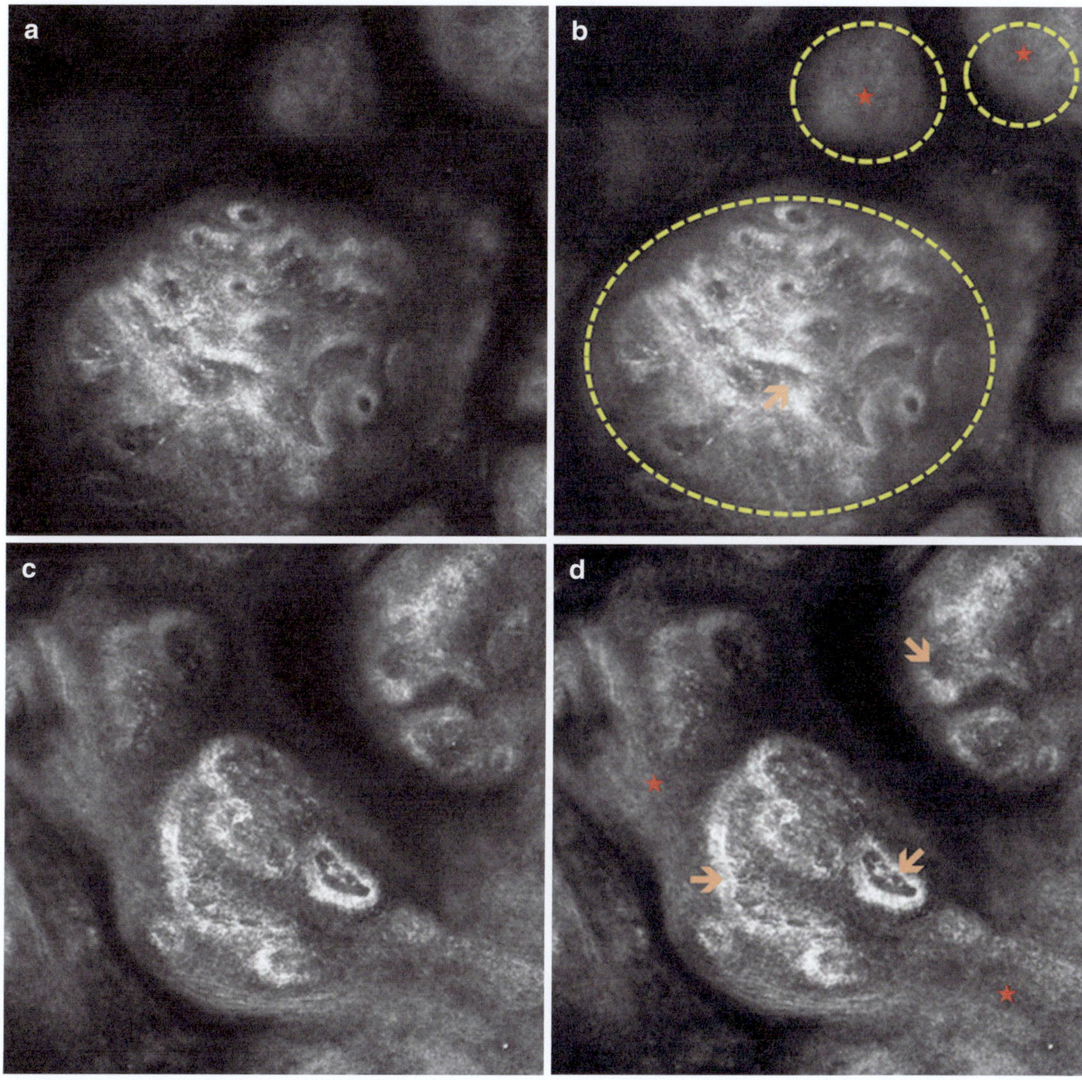

Fig. 4.11 IVCM features of common form of seborrheic keratosis (**a**–**d**)

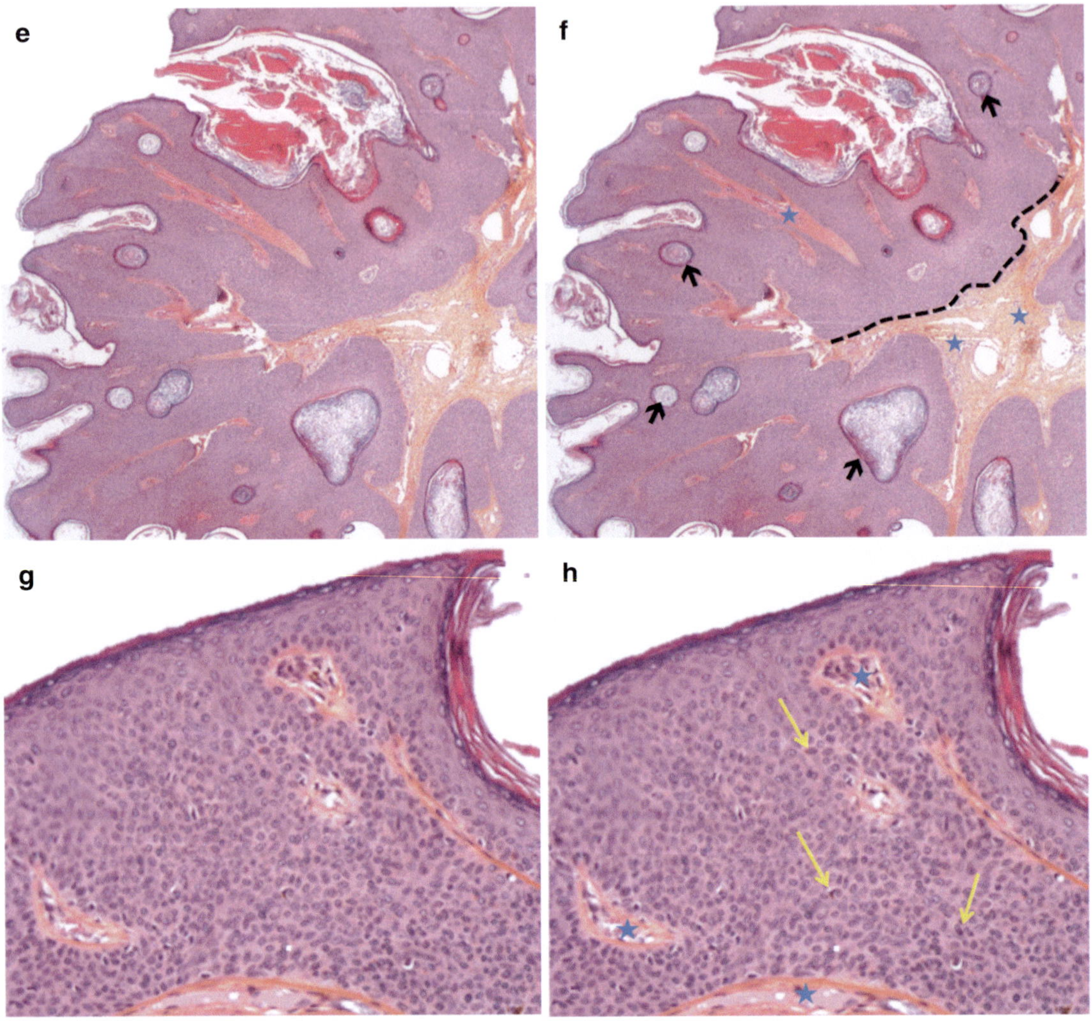

Fig. 4.12 Histological features of common form of seborrheic keratosis (**e–h**). (**e**, **f**) ×25 HES. (**g**, **h**) ×100 HES

4.4.2 Seborrheic Keratosis: Hyperkeratotic Form

The clinical aspect (Fig. 4.13) is that of a hyperkeratotic pedunculated lesion, most often pigmented.

The IVCM features are as follows (Fig. 4.14a–d):

- Acanthotic epidermis (*red stars*) with regular honeycomb pattern and hyperkeratosis can be seen. No abnormal cells are seen.
- Horny pseudocysts in the epidermis containing keratotic hyperreflective debris (*green arrows*).
- Dermo-epidermal junction in the form of irregular bright rings (polycyclic papillary contours) bordered by small bright cells (*orange circle*).
- Superficial dermis consisting of normal and bright plump cells corresponding to melanophages can be seen (*yellow arrows*).

On optical microscopy (Fig. 4.15e–h) the epidermal proliferation is papillomatous with orthokeratotic hyperkeratosis (*green stars*).

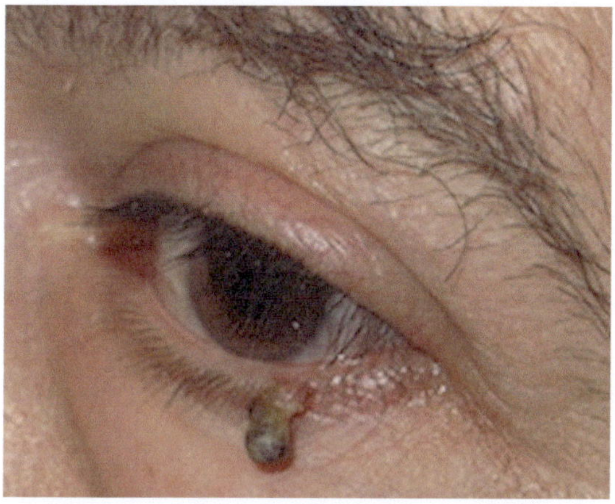

Fig. 4.13 Clinical aspect of hyperkeratotic form of seborrheic keratosis

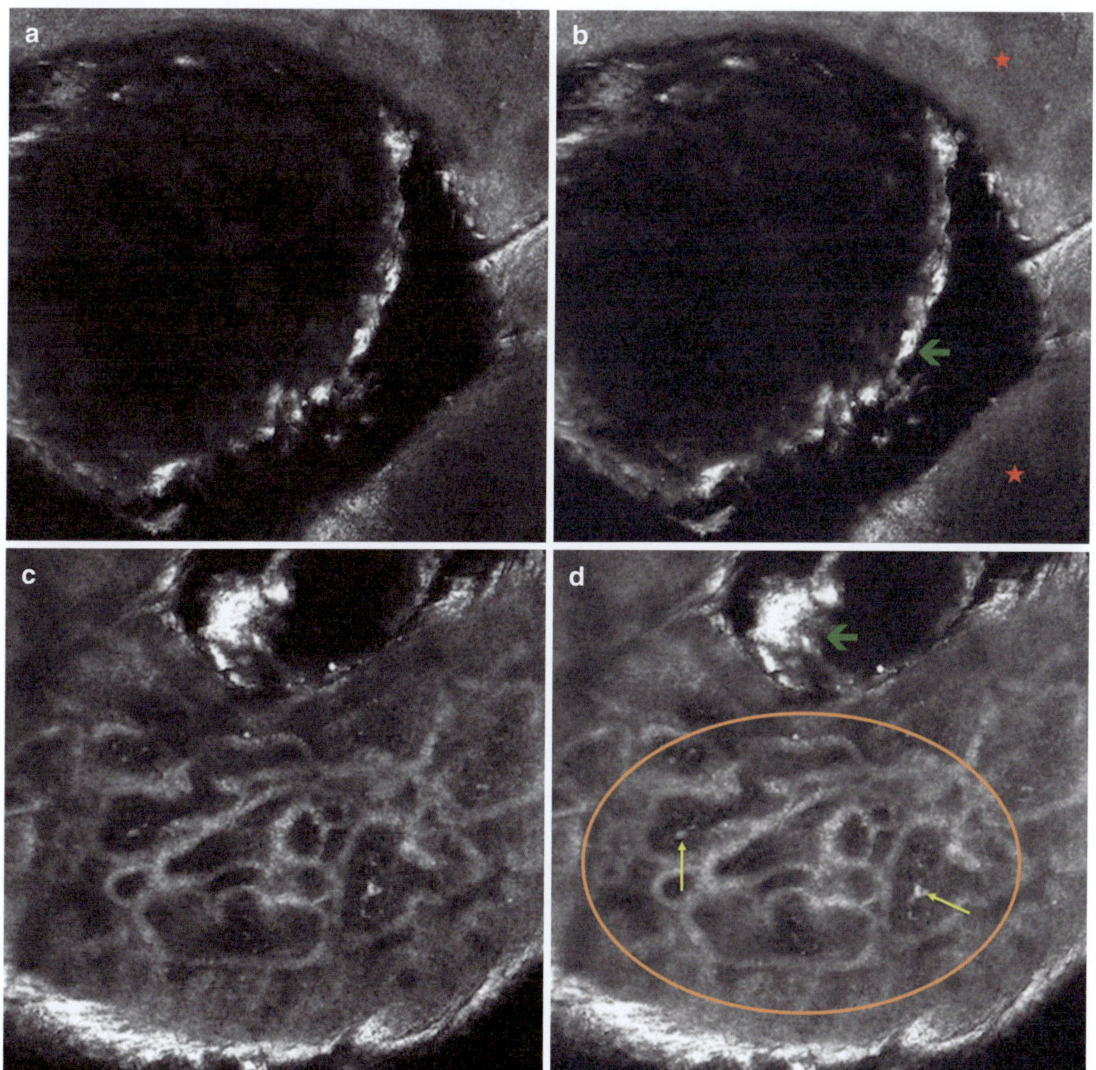

Fig. 4.14 IVCM features of hyperkeratotic form of seborrheic keratosis (**a–d**)

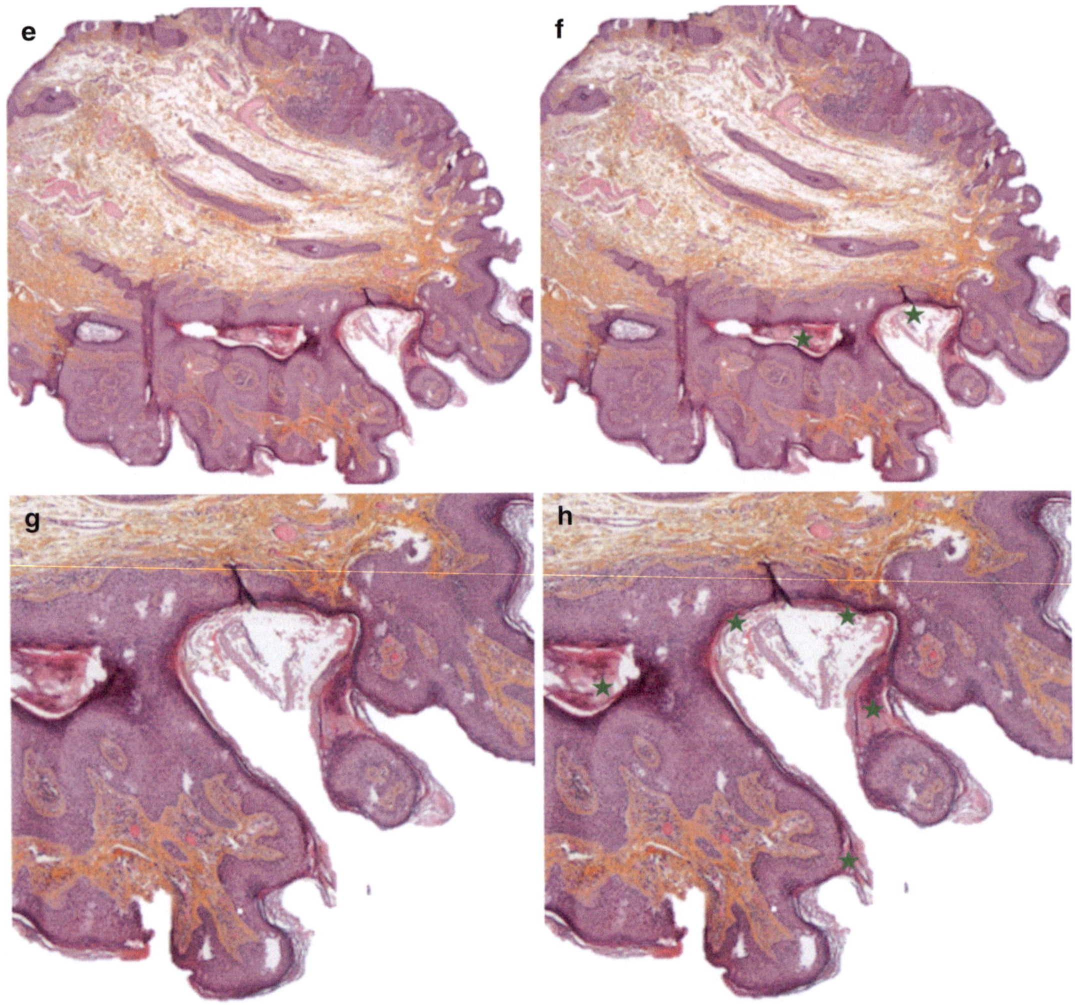

Fig. 4.15 Histological features of hyperkeratotic form of seborrheic keratosis (**e–h**). (**e**, **f**) ×25 HES. (**g**, **h**) ×50 HES

4.4.3 Seborrheic Keratosis: Reticulated Form

The clinical aspect is similar to that of the other histological types of seborrheic keratosis. Here, the shown case (Fig. 4.16a, b) of reticulated seborrheic keratosis is a flat pigmented lesion at the free edge of the right lower eyelid.

The IVCM features are as follows (Fig. 4.17c, d):

- Epidermal proliferation arranged in a fine anastomotic reticulated network.
- Horny pseudocysts (*yellow arrows*).
- Inflammatory cells (melanophages, lymphocytes, and/or Langerhans cells) are prominent in the irritated form of seborrheic keratosis, but they can also be found in the other histological forms of seborrheic keratosis. The present case shows dendritic cells (large irregular, elongated, or triangular bright cells) (*blue arrow*) corresponding to Langerhans cells and scattered lymphocytes (visible as small bright points).
- Superficial dermis is normal.

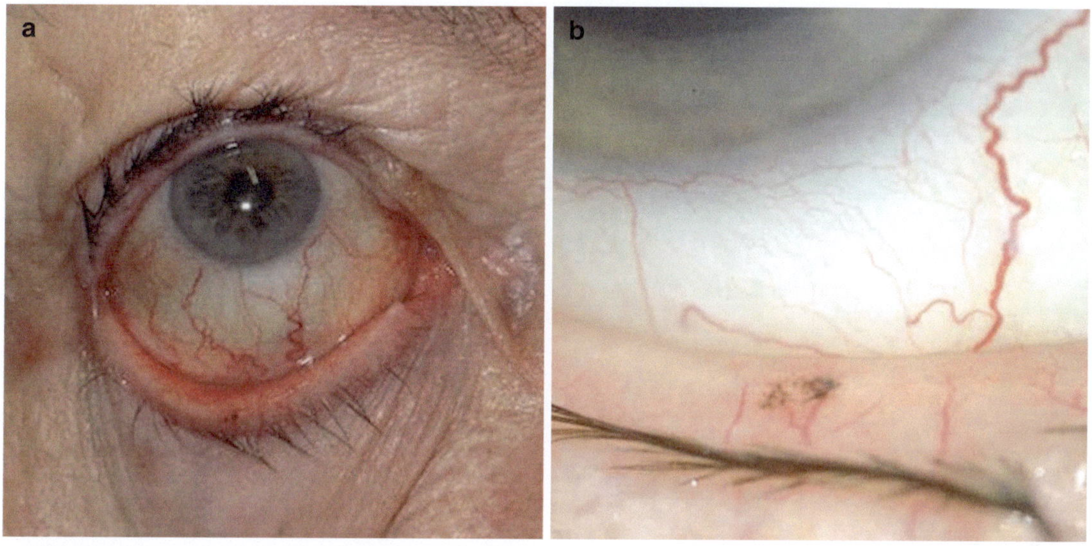

Fig. 4.16 Clinical aspect of reticulated form of seborrheic keratosis: macroscopic photography (**a**), and slit-lamp photography (**b**)

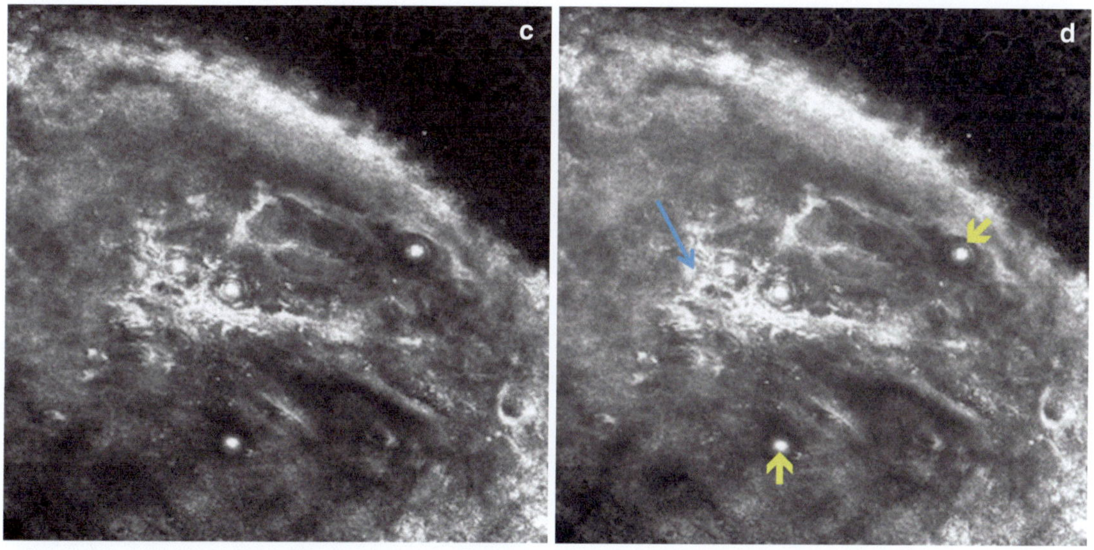

Fig. 4.17 IVCM features of reticulated form of seborrheic keratosis (**c**, **d**)

On optical microscopy the histologic features are as follows (Fig. 4.18e–h):

- At low magnification (e, f), epidermal proliferation is arranged in a fine anastomotic reticulated network that encloses in its meshes islands of dermal connective tissue and horny pseudocysts (*yellow arrows*).
- At high magnification (g, h), epithelial hyperplasia is made up of basaloid cells that are sometimes pigmented (*black dotted line*).

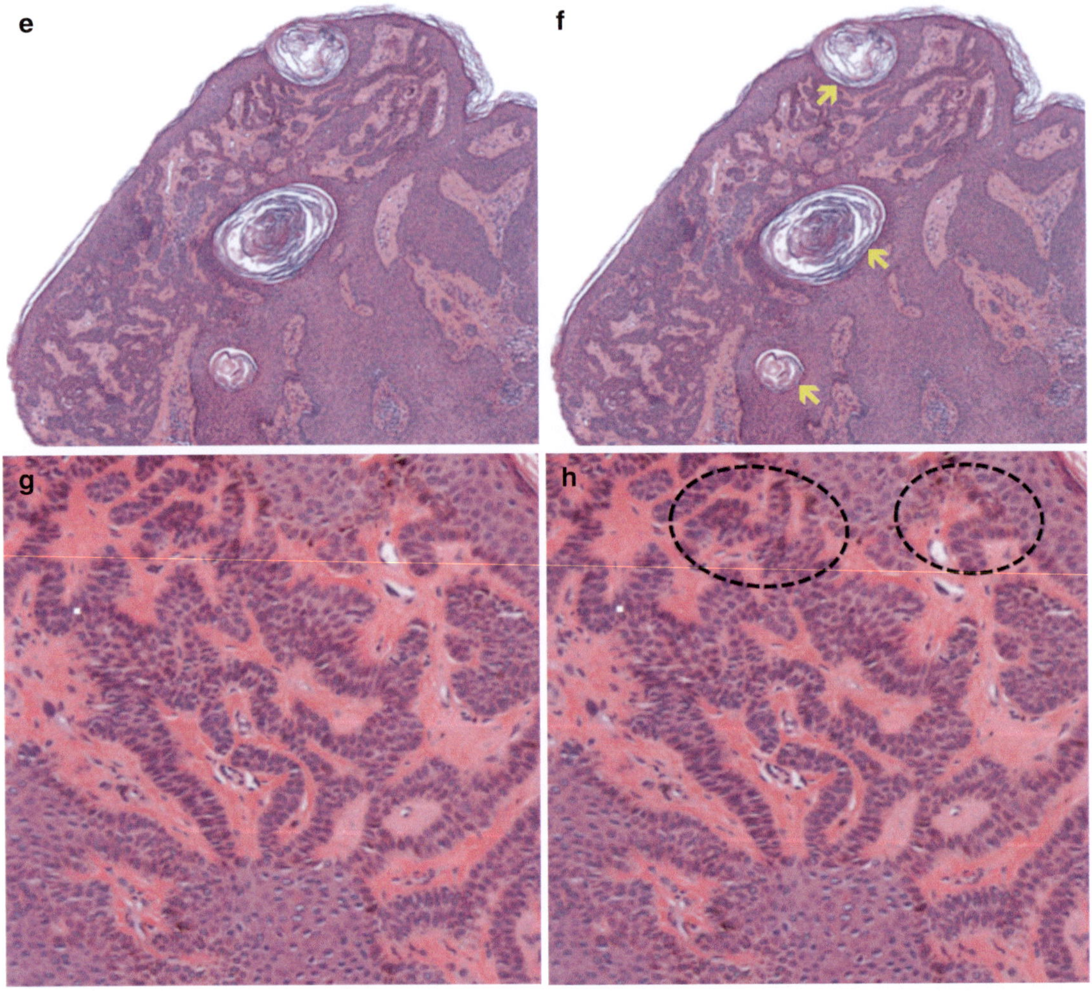

Fig. 4.18 Histological features of reticulated form of seborrheic keratosis (**e**–**h**). (**e**, **f**) ×50 HES. (**g**, **h**) ×100 HES

4.5 Melanoacanthoma

Melanoacanthoma is a rare tumor, mostly located on the face. It is most often unique and pigmented. Clinical diagnosis is difficult because of its similarity to seborrheic keratosis and melanoma.

The present patient has a nevus and melanoacanthoma (*black arrow*) of the free edge of the left lower eyelid (Fig. 4.19). This melanoacanthoma appeared as a reddish macule with irregular margins.

The IVCM features are as follows (Fig. 4.20a–d):

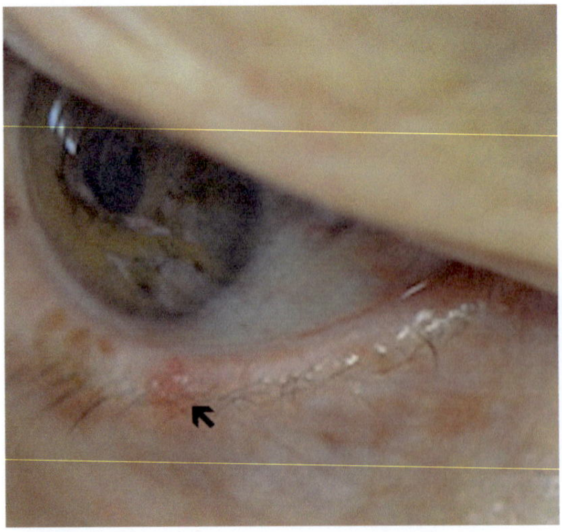

Fig. 4.19 Clinical aspect of melanoacanthoma

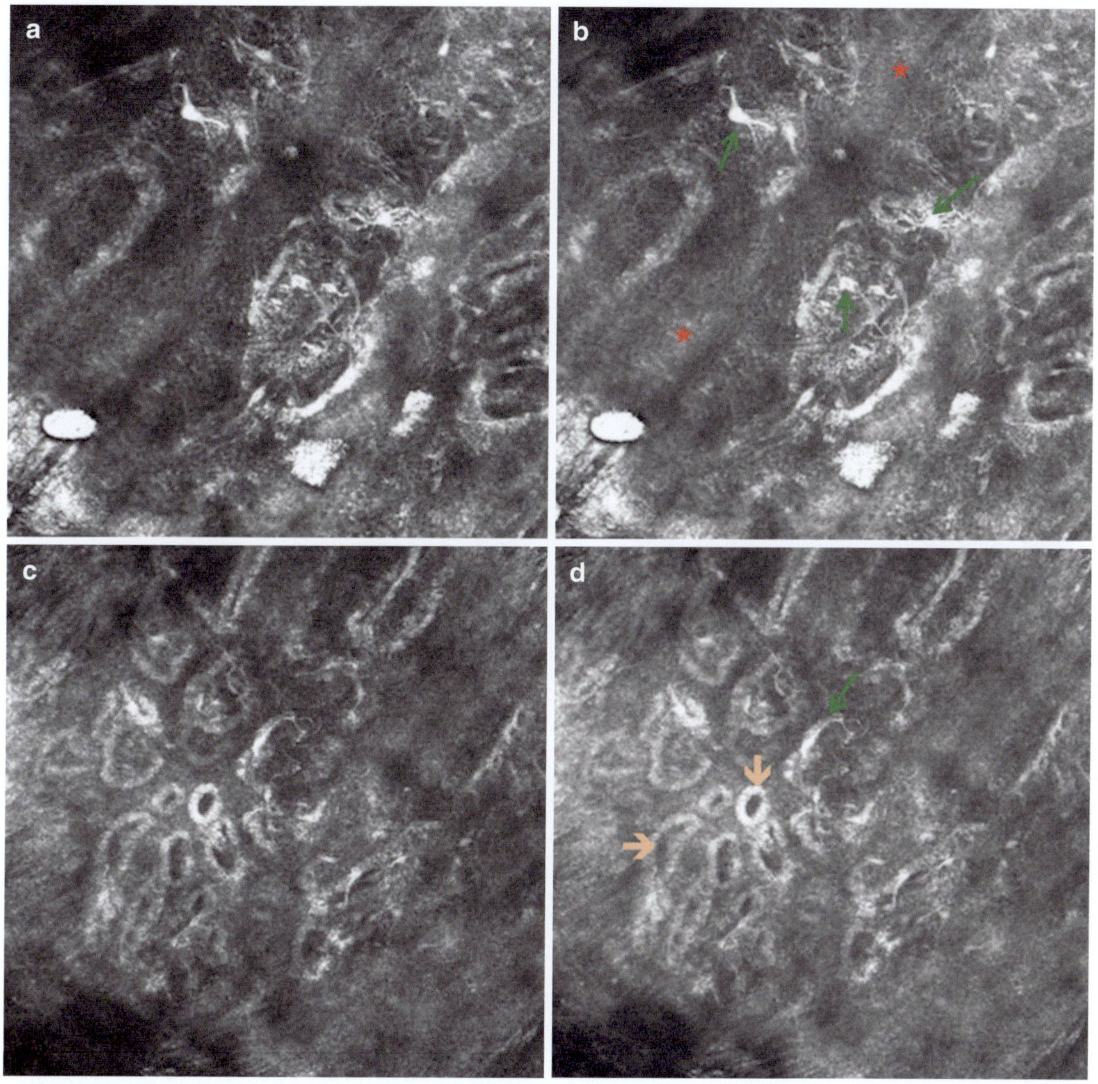

Fig. 4.20 IVCM features of melanoacanthoma (**a**–**d**)

- Regular honeycombed epidermis (*red stars*) with widespread proliferation of homogeneous hyperreflective dendritic cells (*green arrows*) (a, b)
- Dermo-epidermal junction (c, d) in the form of stretched rings bordered by bright cells (*orange arrows*) with some hyperreflective dendritic cells (*green arrows*)

On optical microscopy the histologic features are as follows (Fig. 4.21e–j):

- At low magnification (e, f), epidermal proliferation mimics that of seborrheic keratosis (*black dotted line*). However, proliferation of melanocytes is also present and can be revealed in red by the anti-Melan-A antibody.
- At high magnification (g–j), squamous eddies (*blue arrows*) are present in the acanthotic epithelium. A superficial inflammatory dermal infiltrate is visible (*black stars*). There is an absence of abnormal mitosis.

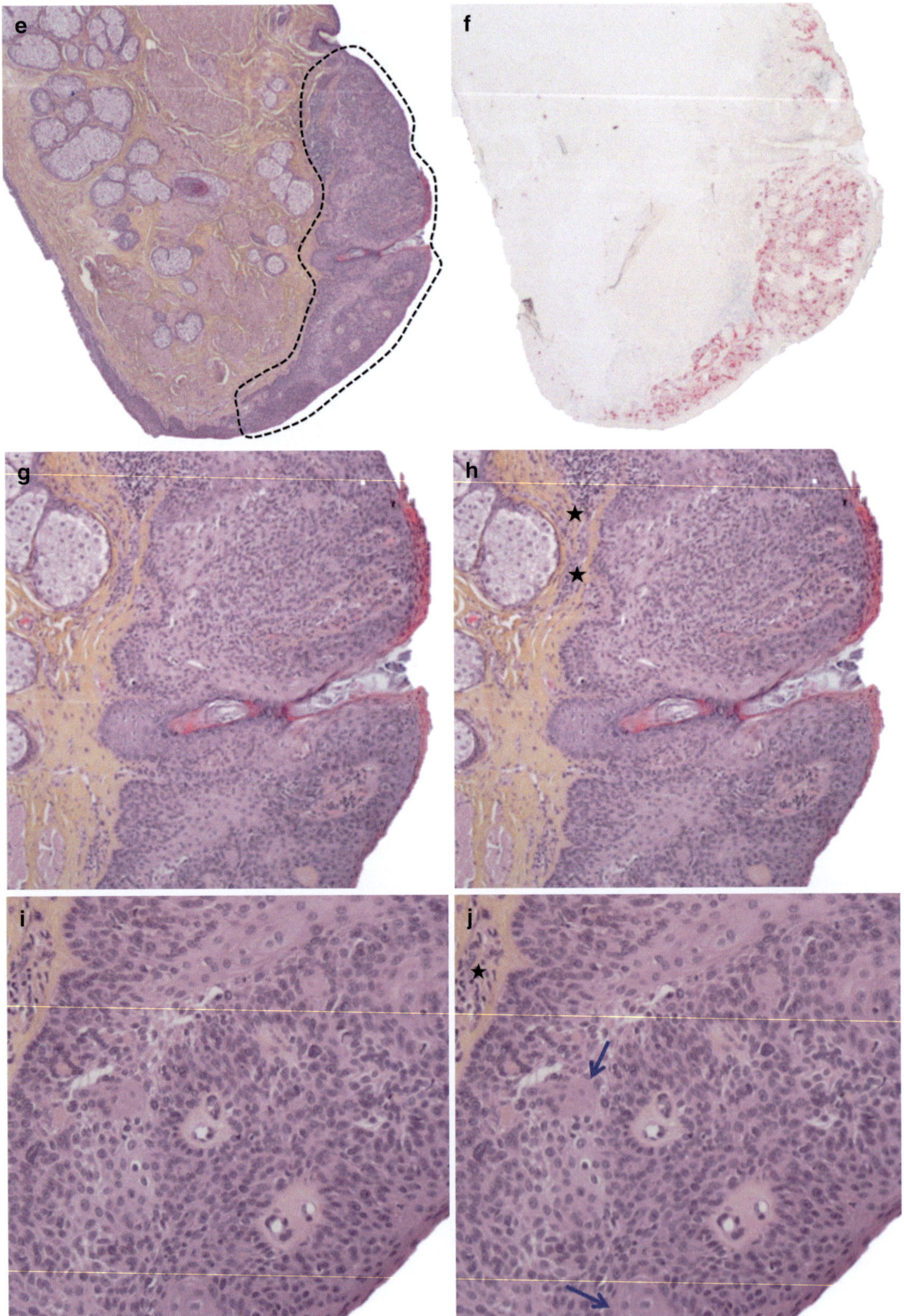

Fig. 4.21 Histological features of melanoacanthoma (**e**–**j**). (**e**) ×25 HES. (**f**) ×25 Anti-Melan-A Ab. (**g**, **h**) ×100 HES. (**i**, **j**) ×200 HES

4.6 Epidermal Cyst

Epidermal cyst can occur at any age but is more common in adolescents or young adults.

The clinical aspect (Fig. 4.22) is a flesh or yellowish cyst measuring a few millimeters to a few centimeters. The milium grain is a small epidermal cyst measuring less than 5 mm in diameter. Its evolution can be inflammatory in case of rupture of its wall.

The IVCM features are as follows (Fig. 4.23a–d):

- Normal epidermis (not shown here).
- Hyporeflective cystic cavity in the superficial dermis filled with keratin (*orange arrows*) and surrounded by a normal epithelium. Keratin

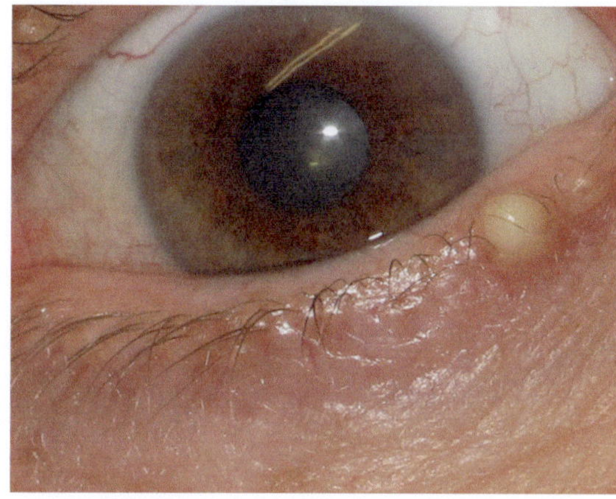

Fig. 4.22 Clinical aspect of epidermal cyst

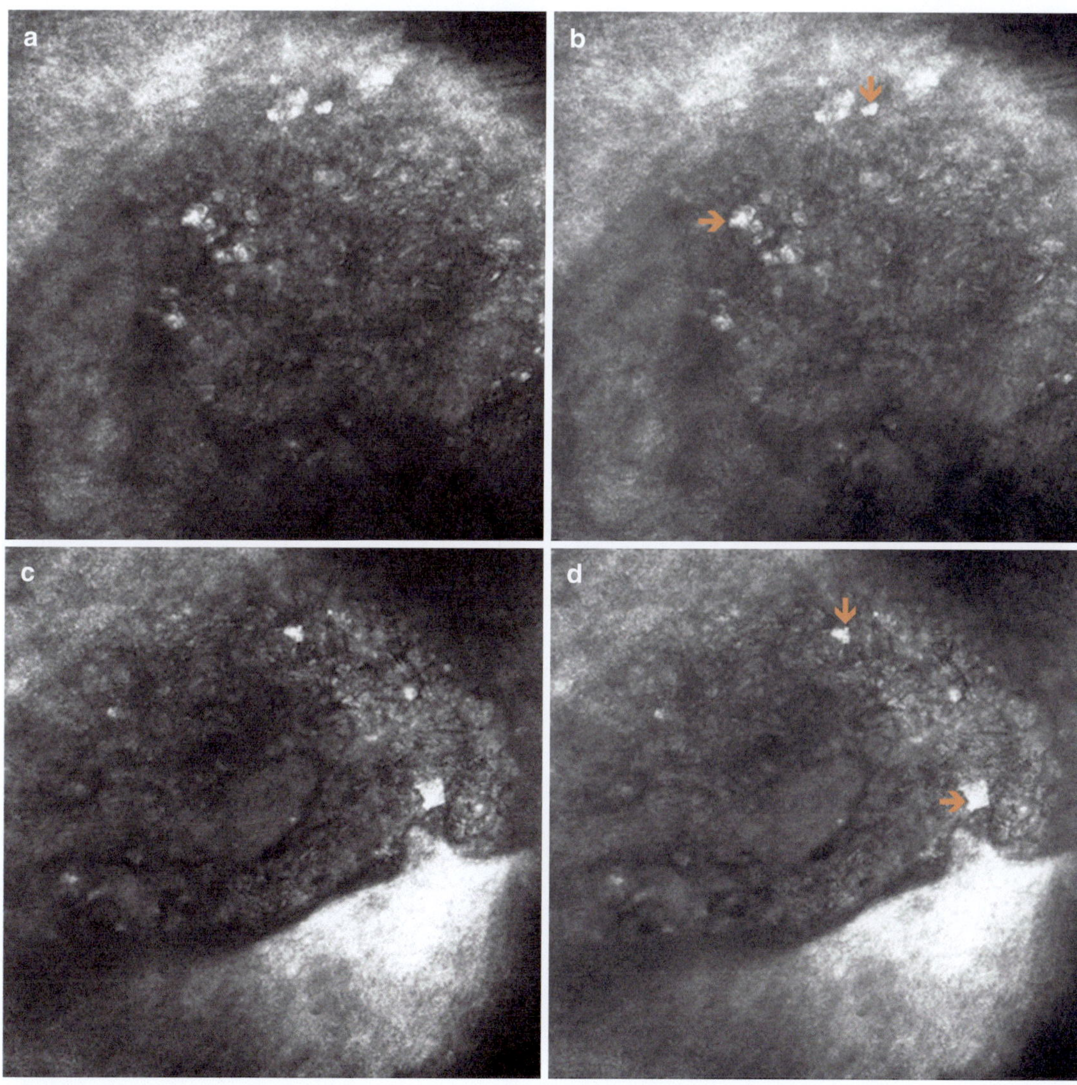

Fig. 4.23 IVCM features of epidermal cyst (**a**–**d**)

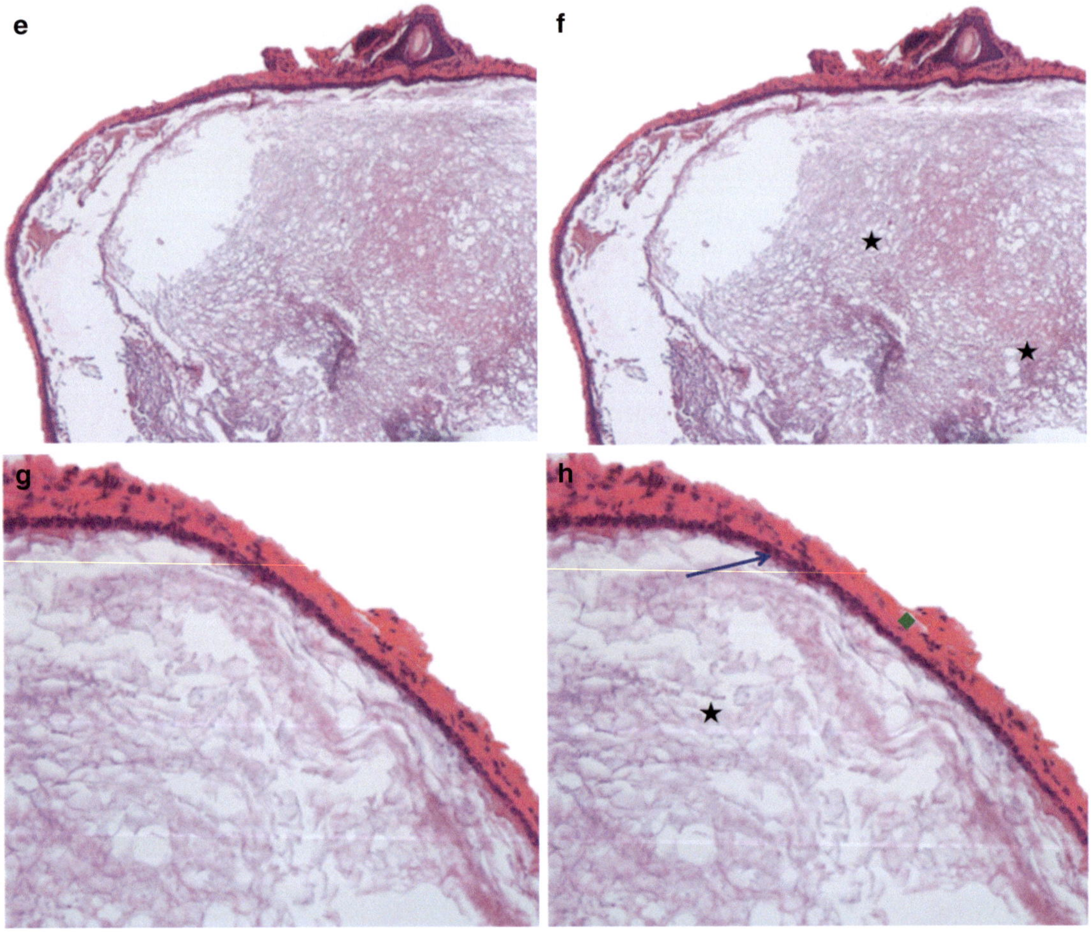

Fig. 4.24 Histological features of epidermal cyst (**e**–**h**). (**e**, **f**) ×25 HES. (**g**, **h**) ×200 HES

(*orange arrows*) is hyperreflective and has a lamellar structure.

On optical microscopy the histologic features are as follows (Fig. 4.24e–h):

– At low magnification (e, f), the cystic lesion is of dermal site, has a thin wall, and is filled of lamellar keratin of laminated appearance (*black stars*).
– At high magnification (g, h), the wall is covered by a normal epidermis (*green diamond*) with a visible granular base (*blue arrow*).

Precancerous Epidermal Lesions

5

Mathilde Kaspi, Thibaud Garcin, Cyril Habougit,
Damien Grivet, Elisa Cinotti, Fabien Forest,
and Jean-Luc Perrot

Content

Abbreviations

Ab	Antibodies
HES	Hematoxylin-eosin-saffron stain
IVCM	In vivo reflectance confocal microscopy

M. Kaspi (✉) · T. Garcin · D. Grivet
Department of Ophthalmology, University Hospital of Saint-Etienne, Saint-Etienne Cedex 2, France
e-mail: mathilde.kaspi@gmail.com; garcinthibaud@gmail.com; damien.grivet@chu-st-etienne.fr

C. Habougit · F. Forest
Department of Pathology, University Hospital of Saint-Etienne, Saint-Etienne Cedex 2, France
e-mail: cyril.habougit@chu-st-etienne.fr; fabien.forest@chu-st-etienne.fr

E. Cinotti
Department of Dermatology, University of Siena, S. Maria alle Scotte Hospital, Siena, Italy
e-mail: elisa.cinotti@unisi.it

J.-L. Perrot
Department of Dermatology, University Hospital of Saint-Etienne, Saint-Etienne Cedex 2, France
e-mail: j.luc.perrot@chu-st-etienne.fr

© Springer Nature Switzerland AG 2020
M. Kaspi et al. (eds.), *Eyelid and Conjunctival Tumors*,
https://doi.org/10.1007/978-3-030-36606-3_5

5.1 Actinic Keratosis

On clinical examination, actinic keratosis is an erythematous and squamous lesion (Fig. 5.1). It typically occurs in photo-exposed areas, hence its name solar or actinic keratosis. It has mild-to-moderate squamous cell dysplasia (low-grade intraepithelial neoplasia). The evolution into squamous cell carcinoma is possible.

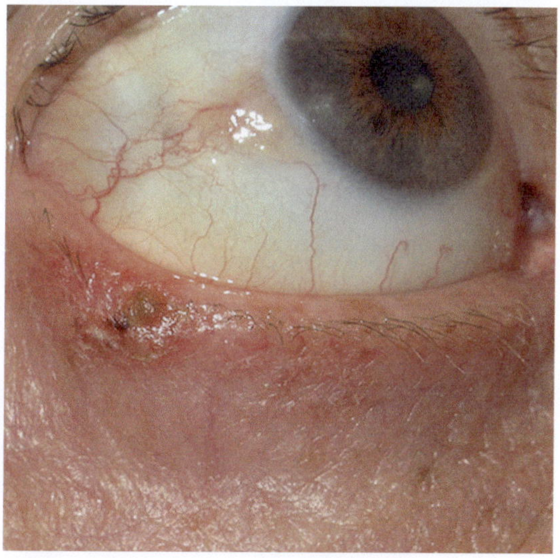

Fig. 5.1 Clinical aspect of actinic keratosis

The IVCM features are as follows (Fig. 5.2a–d):

- Parakeratosis and hyperkeratosis of the stratum corneum of the epidermis (not shown here)
- Irregular honeycomb pattern of the spinous-granular layer of the epidermis or completely disorganized epidermis with large dyskeratotic cells (*light grey circles*)

On optical microscopy the histologic features are as follows (Fig. 5.3e–j):

- At low magnification (e–h), epidermis with hyperkeratosis, parakeratosis (*blue arrows*), and continuous basal membrane (*black line*) is seen. The superficial dermis contains an inflammatory infiltrate (*black stars*). The anti-p53 antibody strongly stains the cells of basal layer in brown (*red diamond*).
- At high magnification (i, j), the epidermis contains cytonuclear atypia in its basal layer without total disorganization of its architecture. The basal membrane is respected (*black line*).

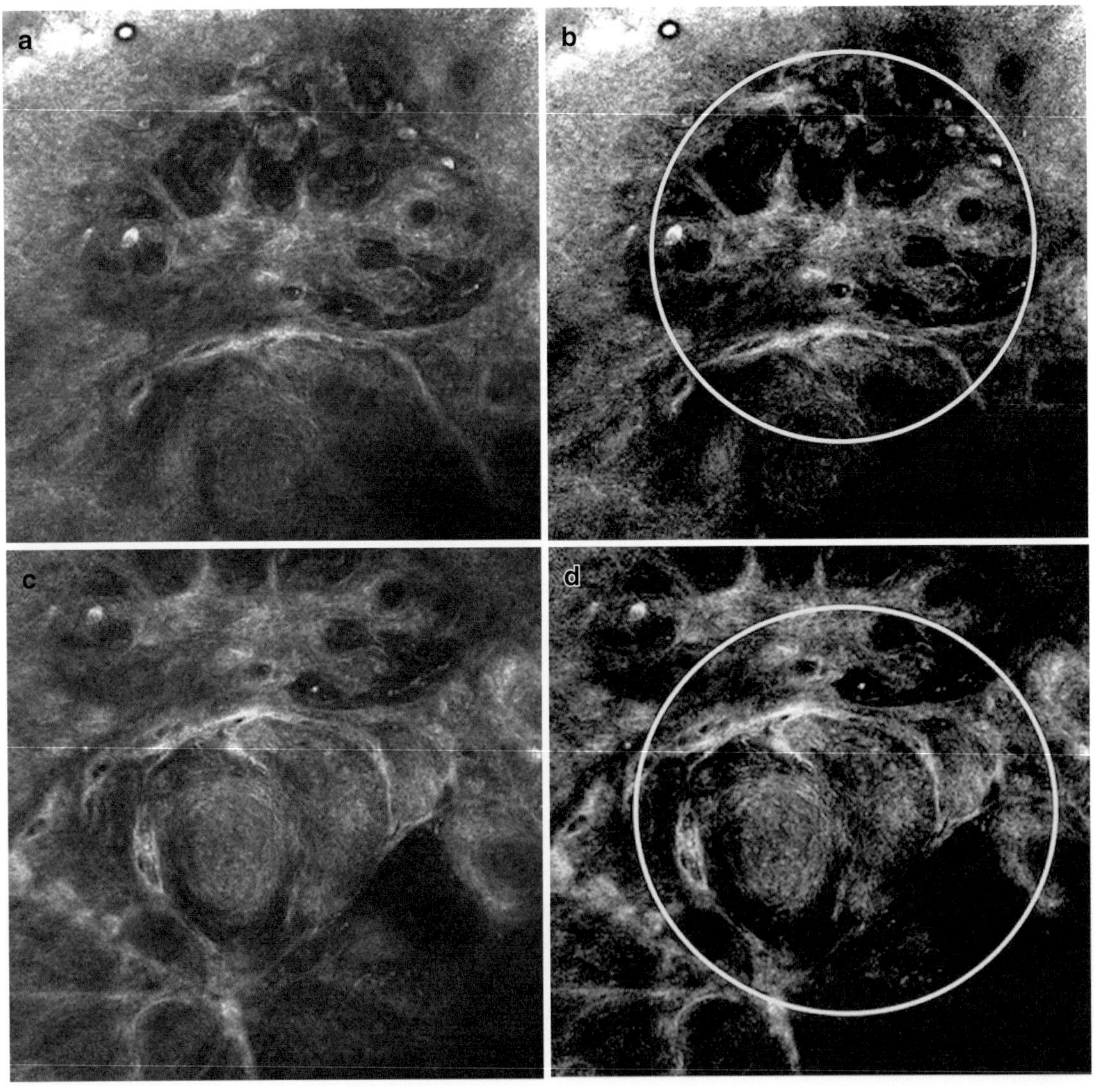

Fig. 5.2 IVCM features of actinic keratosis (**a**–**d**)

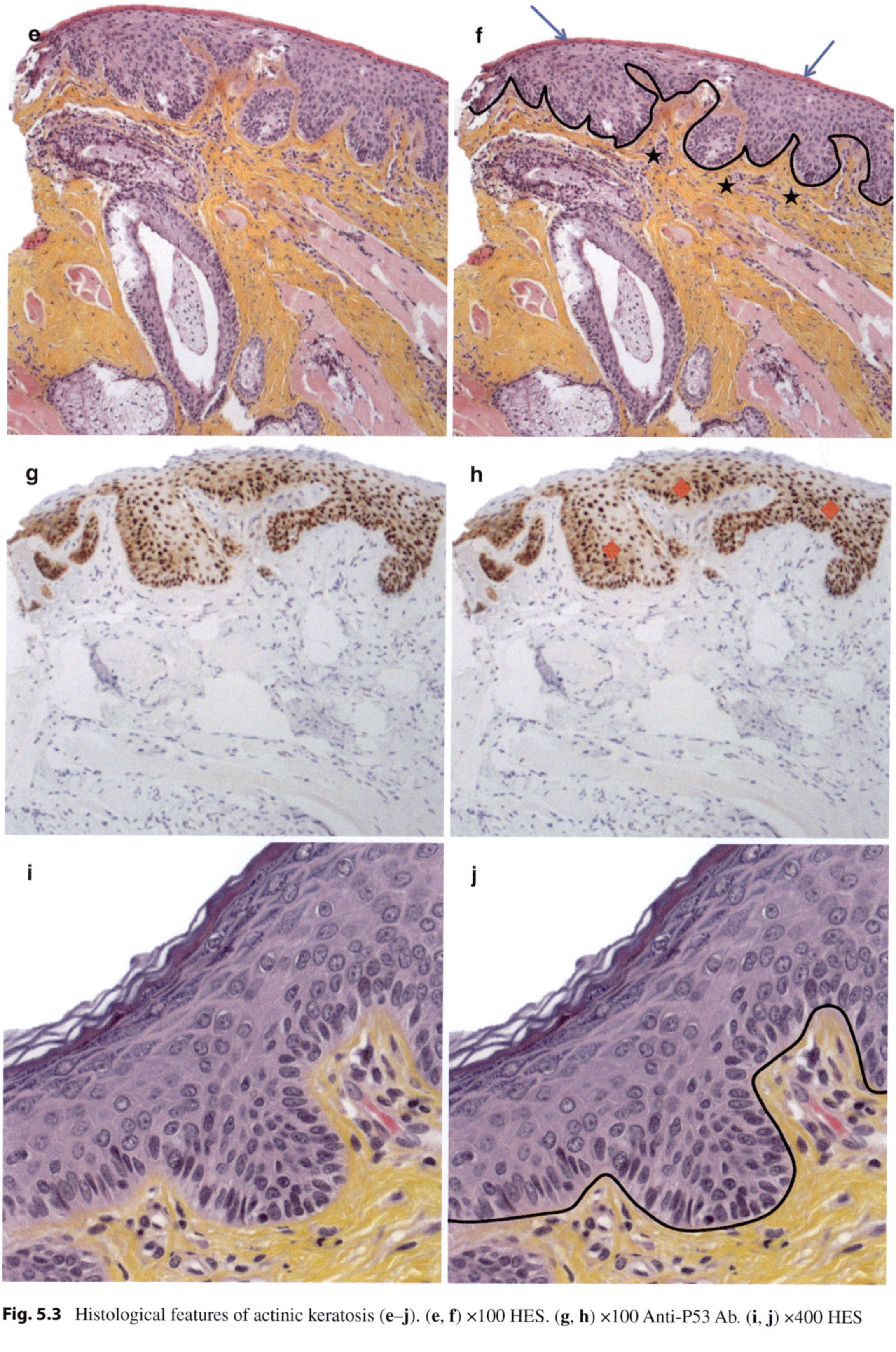

Fig. 5.3 Histological features of actinic keratosis (**e**–**j**). (**e**, **f**) ×100 HES. (**g**, **h**) ×100 Anti-P53 Ab. (**i**, **j**) ×400 HES

Malignant Epidermal Tumors

6

Mathilde Kaspi, Thibaud Garcin, Cyril Habougit, Damien Grivet, Fabien Forest, Jean-Luc Perrot, and Elisa Cinotti

Contents

Abbreviations

HES Hematoxylin-eosin-saffron stain
IVCM In vivo reflectance confocal microscopy

6.1 Squamous Cell Carcinoma

The occurrence of squamous cell carcinoma may be preceded by actinic keratosis or not. Squamous cell carcinoma in situ has the appearance of a clinically well-delineated flat, erythematous, and squamous lesion. Conversely, invasive squamous cell carcinoma is a budding lesion with infiltration of the surrounding normal skin and possible ulceration.

The present patient has an erythematous and ulcerated lesion of the right upper eyelid extending to the outer canthus (Fig. 6.1). Madarosis is present.

M. Kaspi (✉) · T. Garcin · D. Grivet
Department of Ophthalmology, University Hospital of Saint-Etienne, Saint-Etienne Cedex 2, France
e-mail: mathilde.kaspi@gmail.com; garcinthibaud@gmail.com; damien.grivet@chu-st-etienne.fr

C. Habougit · F. Forest
Department of Pathology, University Hospital of Saint-Etienne, Saint-Etienne Cedex 2, France
e-mail: cyril.habougit@chu-st-etienne.fr; fabien.forest@chu-st-etienne.fr

J.-L. Perrot
Department of Dermatology, University Hospital of Saint-Etienne, Saint-Etienne Cedex 2, France
e-mail: j.luc.perrot@chu-st-etienne.fr

E. Cinotti
Department of Dermatology, University of Siena, S. Maria alle Scotte Hospital, Siena, Italy
e-mail: elisa.cinotti@unisi.it

© Springer Nature Switzerland AG 2020
M. Kaspi et al. (eds.), *Eyelid and Conjunctival Tumors*,
https://doi.org/10.1007/978-3-030-36606-3_6

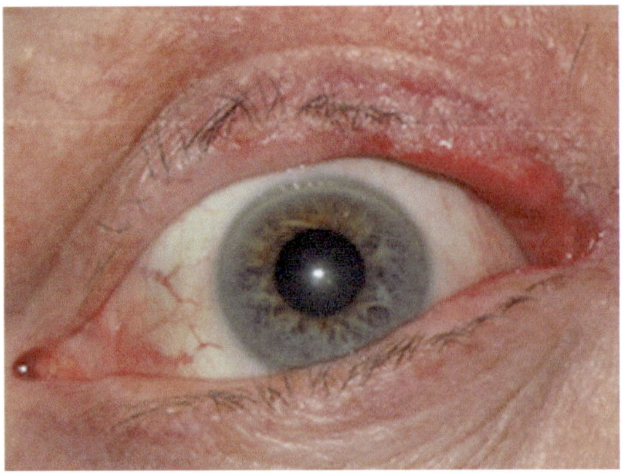

Fig. 6.1 Clinical aspect of squamous cell carcinoma

The IVCM features are as follows (Fig. 6.2a–d):

- Irregular honeycomb pattern or completely disorganized aspect of the epidermis (*yellow stars*) that highly differs from the surrounding normal epidermis with regular honeycomb pattern (*red stars*).
- Two types of targetoid cells can be appreciated in the context of the atypical honeycombed pattern: large cells with a hyperreflective center surrounded by a dark halo and large cells with a dark center and a bright rim and a surrounding dark halo. These

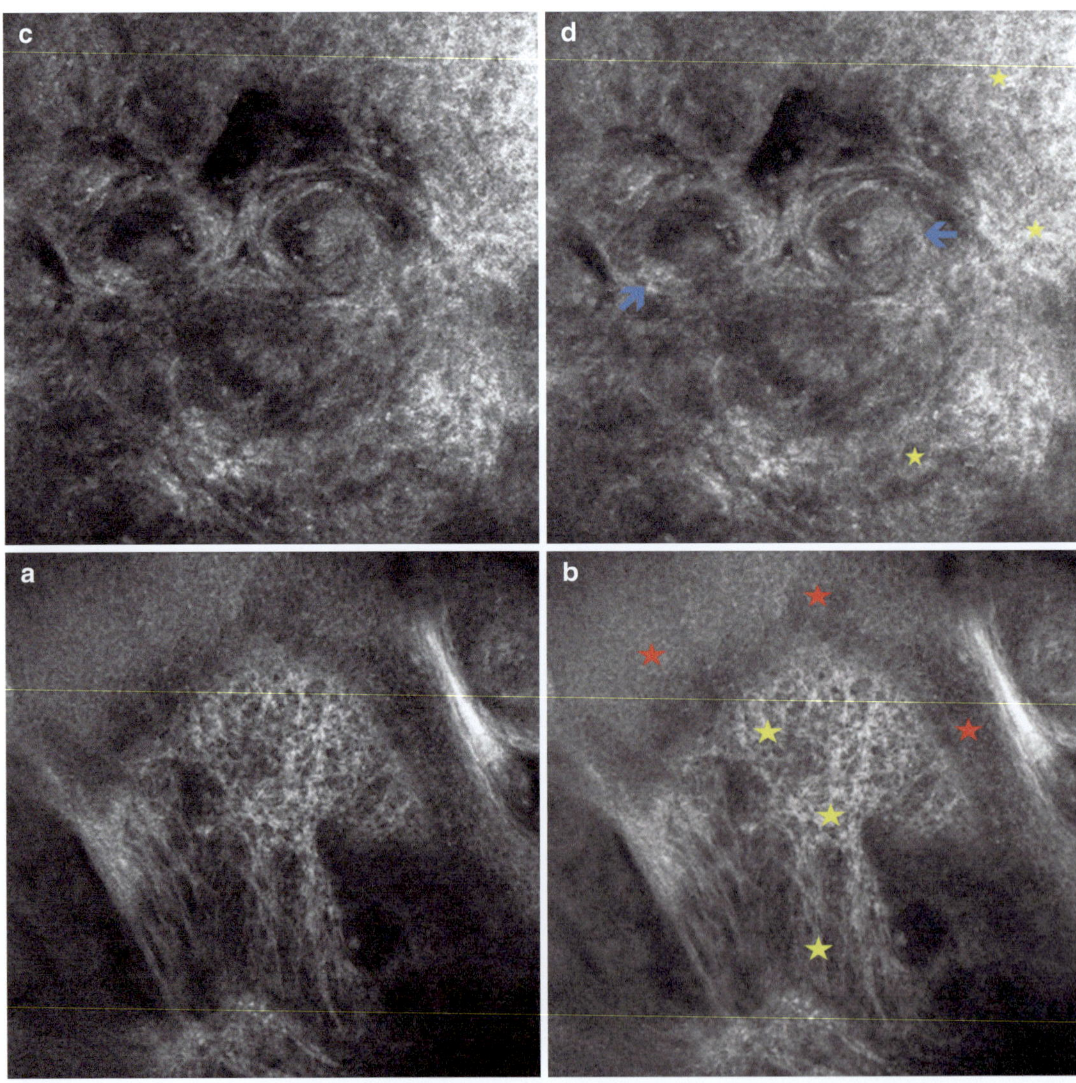

Fig. 6.2 IVCM features of squamous cell carcinoma (**a**–**d**)

cells correspond to dyskeratotic cells at different stages. We observe here clusters of keratinocytes (*blues arrows*).
- Horizontal and dilated blood vessels are sometimes present.

On optical microscopy the histologic features are as follows (Fig. 6.3e–h):

- At low magnification (e, f), atypical squamous cells proliferation is seen involving the whole thickness of the epidermis and disrupting its architecture. These atypical squamous cells cross the basal membrane of the dermo-epidermal junction to infiltrate the dermis in the form of nests or trabeculae (*yellow stars*).
- At high magnification (g, h), differentiation is medium; tumor cells are arranged in small clusters, sometimes around a keratin pearl (*blue arrow*).

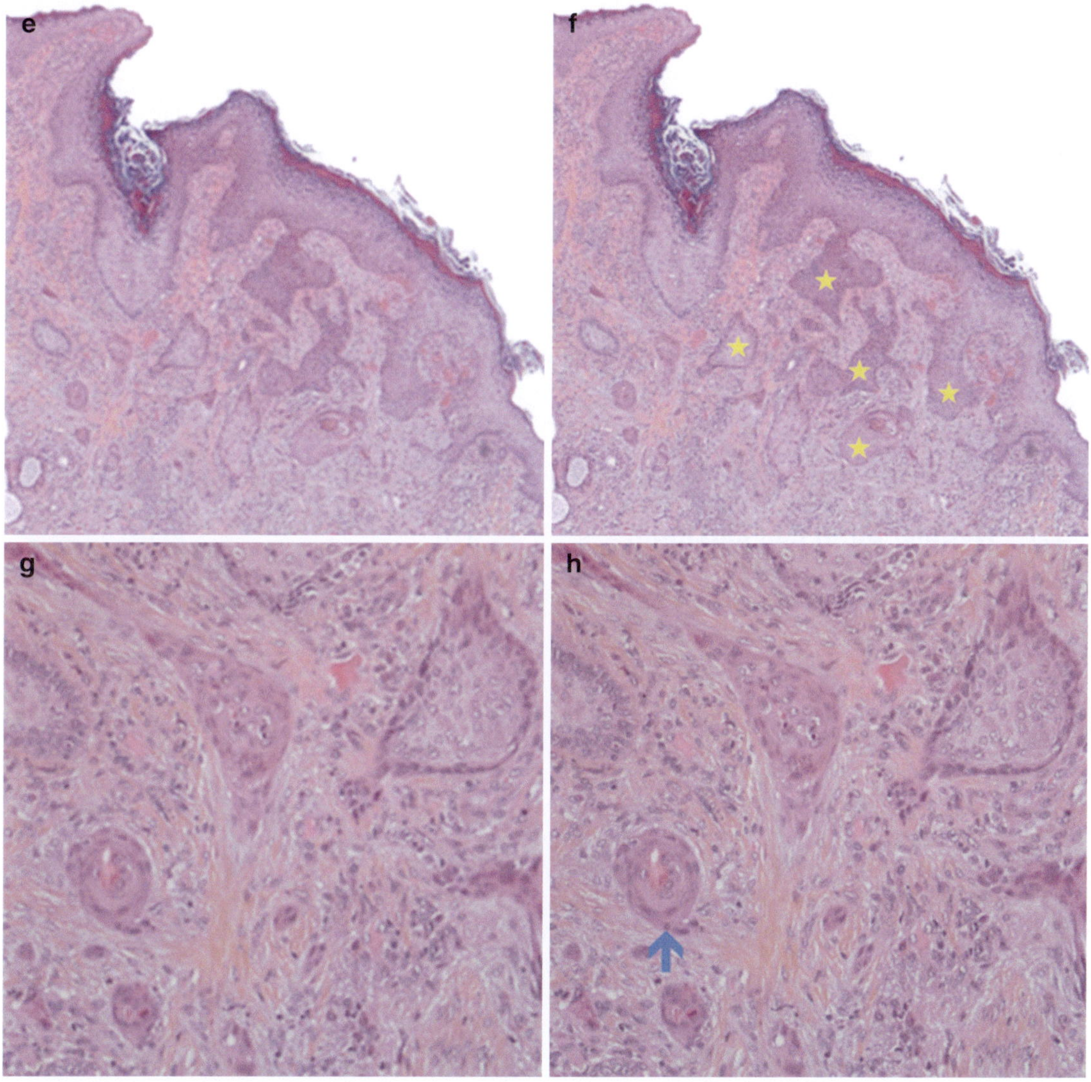

Fig. 6.3 Histological features of squamous cell carcinoma (**e**–**h**). (**e**, **f**) ×50 HES. (**g**, **h**) ×200 HES

6.2 Basal Cell Carcinoma

The main three clinico-histological forms of basal cell carcinoma are nodular, superficial, and infiltrative (or morpheaform or sclerosing).

The diagnosis of basal cell carcinoma in IVCM is very strongly suspected if at least two criteria are present among the following [1, 2]:

- Dark silhouettes, consisting of hyporeflective tumor islands that appear as footprint-like shadow in a context of bright compact collagen and are mainly found in nonpigmented and infiltrative basal cell carcinoma
- Tumor islands of tightly packed weakly to moderately reflective cells with peripheral palisading of elongated cells and oval (lobular nests), elongated, or polycyclic cord-like shape (trabecular structures)
- Peritumoral clefts, corresponding to mucinous stroma
- Convoluted and dilated blood vessels
- Polarized elongated keratinocytes (streaming) of the overlying epidermidis

An inflammatory infiltrate can be found around and inside the islands of basal cell carcinoma (small bright cells corresponding to lymphocytes and neutrophils).

6.2.1 Nodular Basal Cell Carcinoma

The clinical aspect (Fig. 6.4) of nodular basal cell carcinoma is a pearly, translucent lesion with fine telangiectasia on its surface. Madarosis is present. This is the most common clinical form of basal cell carcinoma of the eyelid.

The IVCM features are as follows (Fig. 6.5a–d):

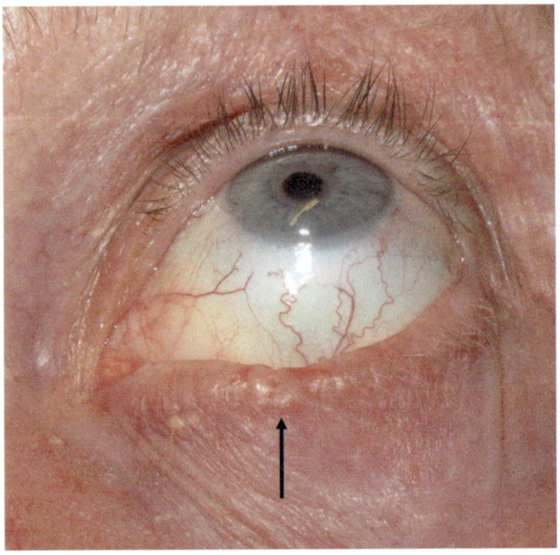

Fig. 6.4 Clinical aspect of nodular basal cell carcinoma

- Normal epidermis of regular honeycomb architecture (not visible here)
- Under the dermo-epidermal junction, lobular nests of tightly packed cells surrounded by peritumoral clefts and hyperreflective stroma or dark silhouettes (*yellow stars*) surrounded by hyperreflective stroma (*green diamonds*).

On optical microscopy the histologic features are as follows (Fig. 6.6e–h):

- At low magnification (e–f), very limited basophilic lobules are grouped together (*black dotted lines*) in the superficial dermis facing stromal retraction.
- At high magnification (g–h), the lobules are composed of basophilic cells, with palisades at the periphery of lobules (*yellow stars*). The cells are densely packed with an oval nucleus and a scarce cytoplasm (*green arrows*).

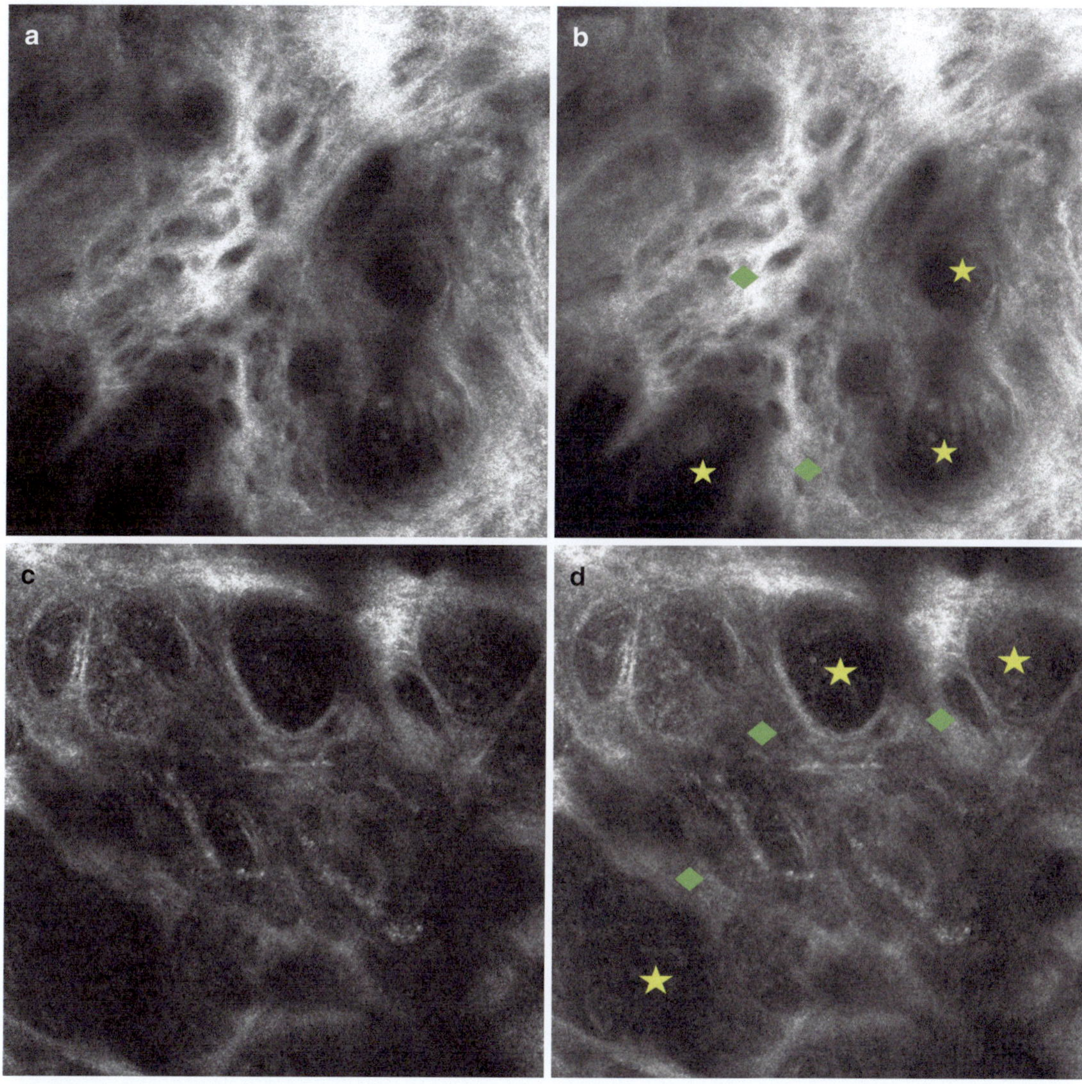

Fig. 6.5 IVCM features of nodular basal cell carcinoma (**a**–**d**)

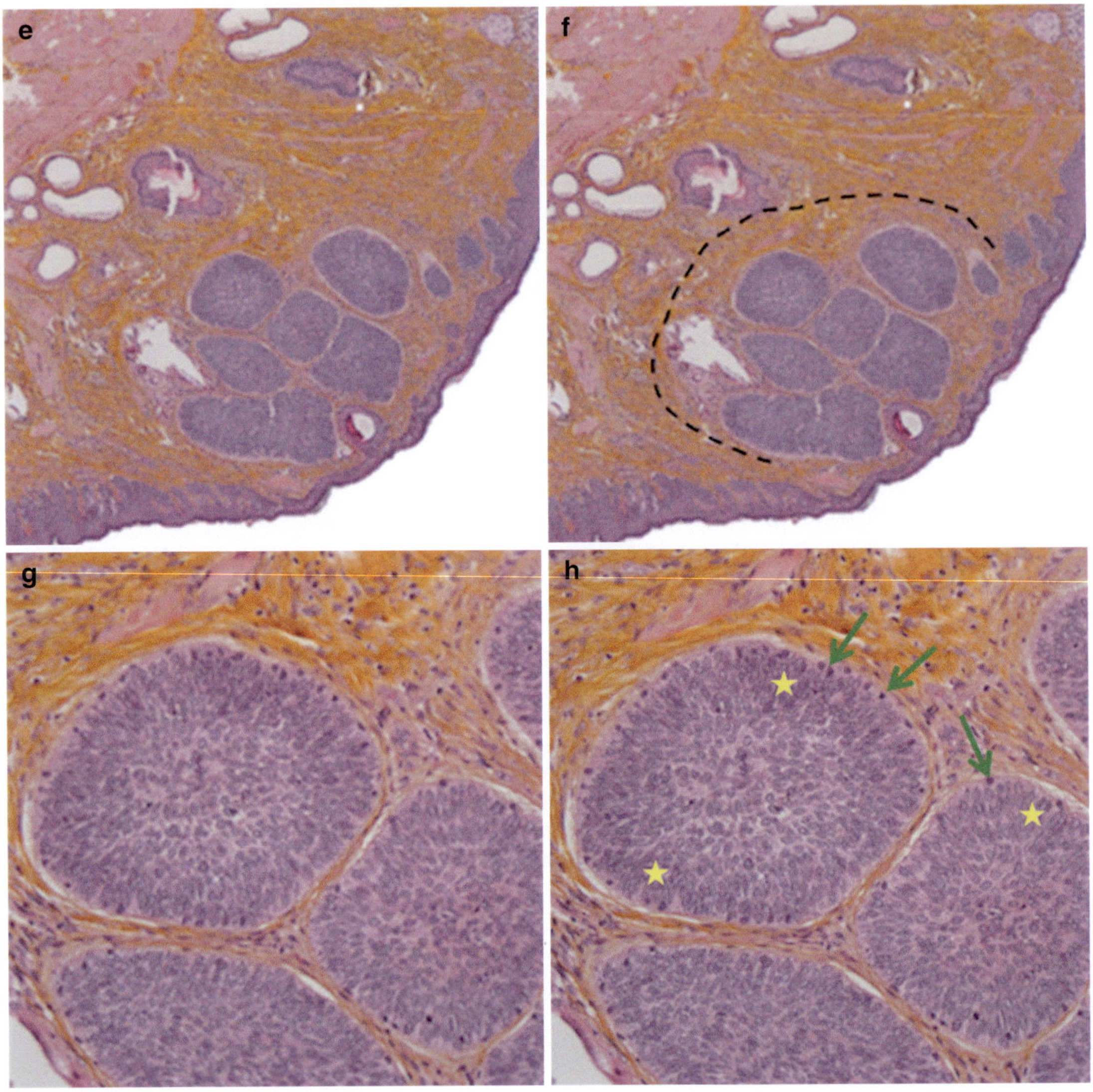

Fig. 6.6 Histological features of nodular basal cell carcinoma (**e**–**h**). (**e**, **f**) ×50 HES. (**g**, **h**) ×200 HES

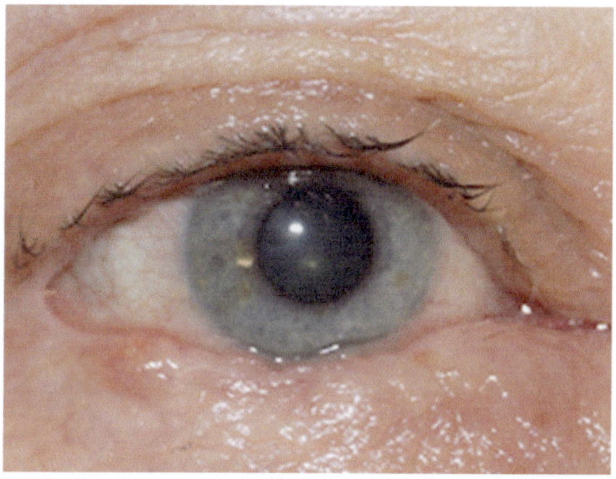

Fig. 6.7 Clinical aspect of superficial basal cell carcinoma

6.2.2 Superficial Basal Cell Carcinoma

The typical clinical appearance (Fig. 6.7) of superficial basal cell carcinoma is an erythematous patch with a possible pearled border. The eyelid margin of the present patient is irregular because she has already had surgery for another basal cell carcinoma of her eyelid.

The IVCM features are as follows (Fig. 6.8a–d):

– Regular honeycombed epidermis (*red stars*) is seen, with polarized elongated keratinocytes.

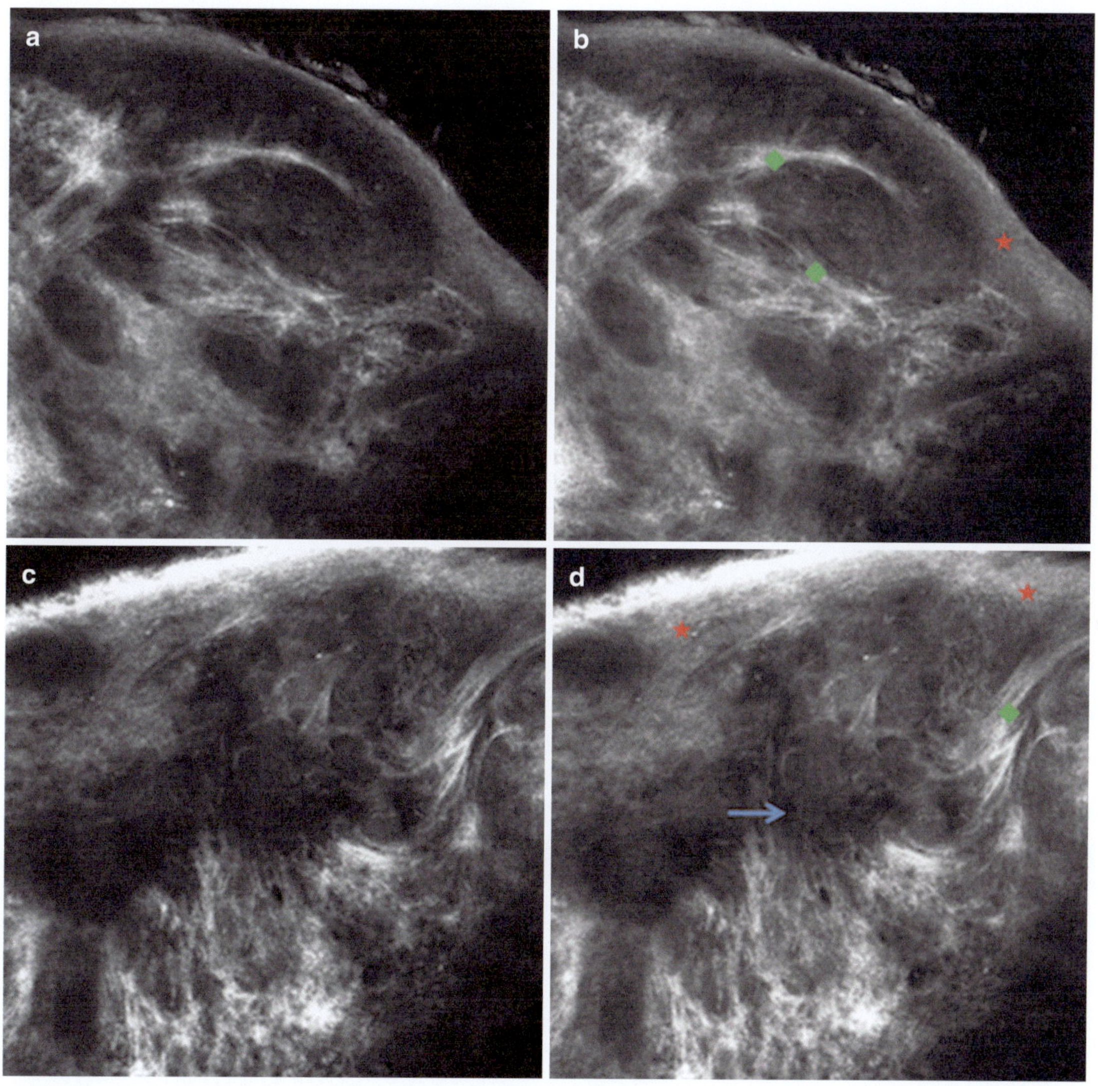

Fig. 6.8 IVCM features of superficial basal cell carcinoma (**a**–**d**)

– Under the dermo-epidermal junction, tumor islands are visible as dark silhouettes (a, b) or islands of moderately reflective cells (c, d) surrounded by hyporeflective peritumoral clefts (*blue arrow*) and hyperreflective collagen (*green diamonds*).

On optical microscopy the histologic features are as follows (Fig. 6.9e–h):

– At low magnification (e, f), tumor clusters are linked to the epidermal basal membrane, taking a garland-like appearance (*black dotted line*).
– At high magnification (g, h), the clusters are composed of basophilic cells with a palisading arrangement of the cells at the periphery (*black arrows*). The underlying dermis contains an inflammatory infiltrate (*blue stars*) (g, h).

6.2.3 Sclerosing Basal Cell Carcinoma

On clinical examination (Fig. 6.10), this subtype of basal cell carcinoma is a whitish, indurated, poorly limited, sometimes retractable plaque (as here), with possible telangiectasias on its surface. Madarosis is present.

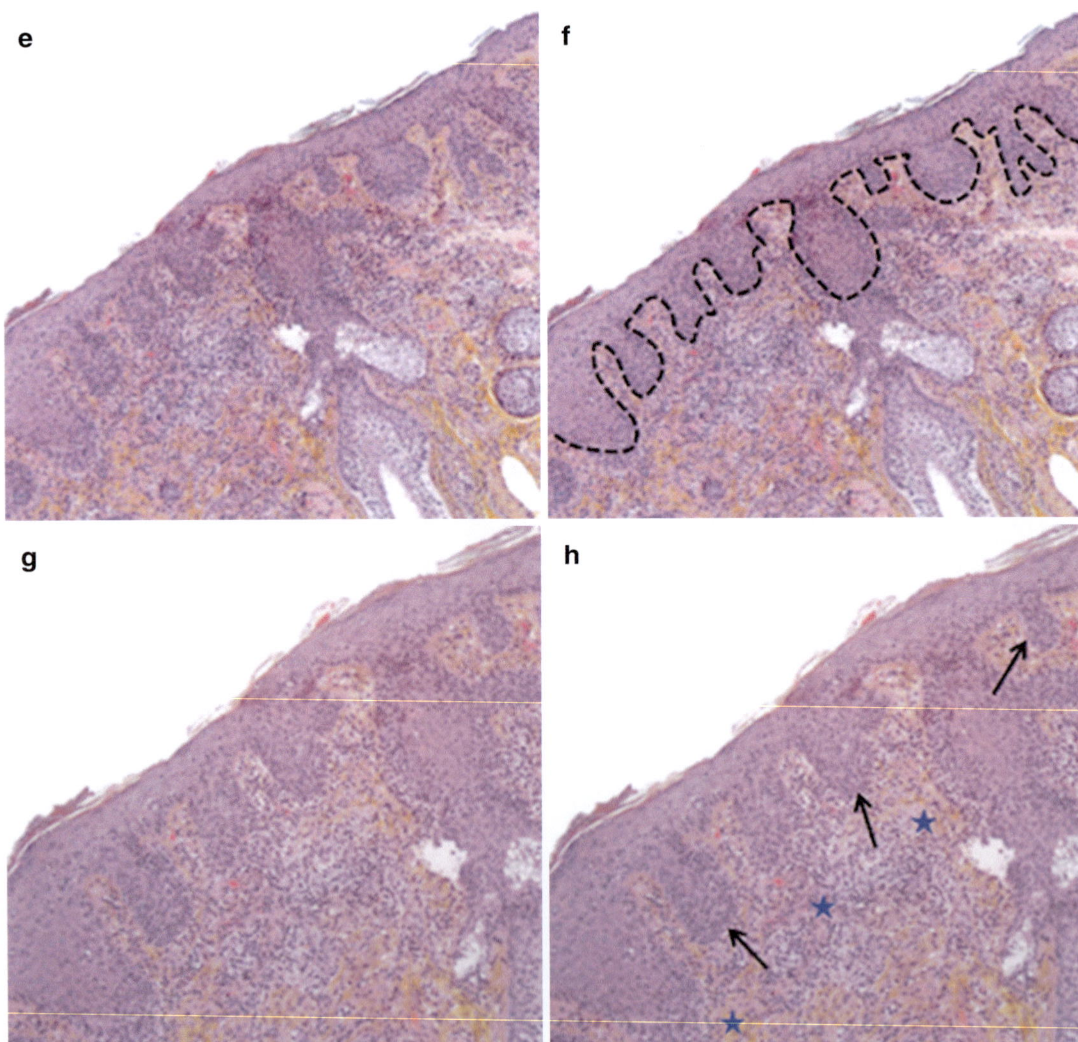

Fig. 6.9 Histological features of superficial basal cell carcinoma (**e**–**h**). (**e**, **f**) ×50 HES. (**g**, **h**) ×100 HES

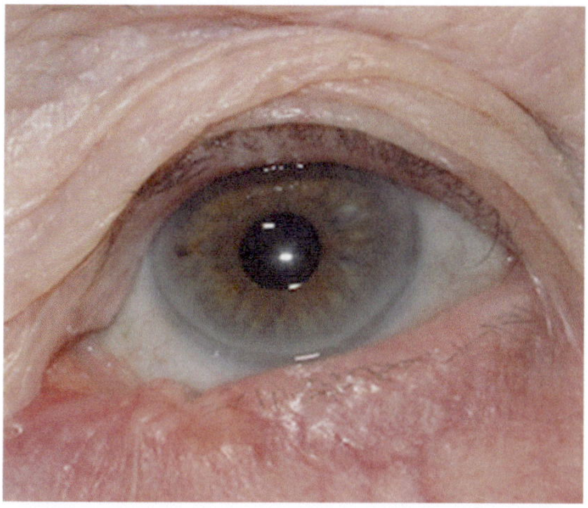

Fig. 6.10 Clinical aspect of sclerosing basal cell carcinoma

On IVCM (Fig. 6.11a–d), under the dermo-epidermal junction, dark silhouettes (*yellow stars*) are surrounded by hyperreflective collagen (*green diamonds*).

On optical microscopy the histologic features are as follows (Fig. 6.12e–j):

- At low magnification (e, f), the proliferation of basophilic cells occurs as stretched thin spans infiltrating the dermis (*black dotted lines*). The epidermis is respected (*blue arrows*).
- At high magnification (g–j), the basophilic cells constituting these spans (*yellow stars*) do not contain a palisade edge. The stroma is fibrous (*green diamonds*).

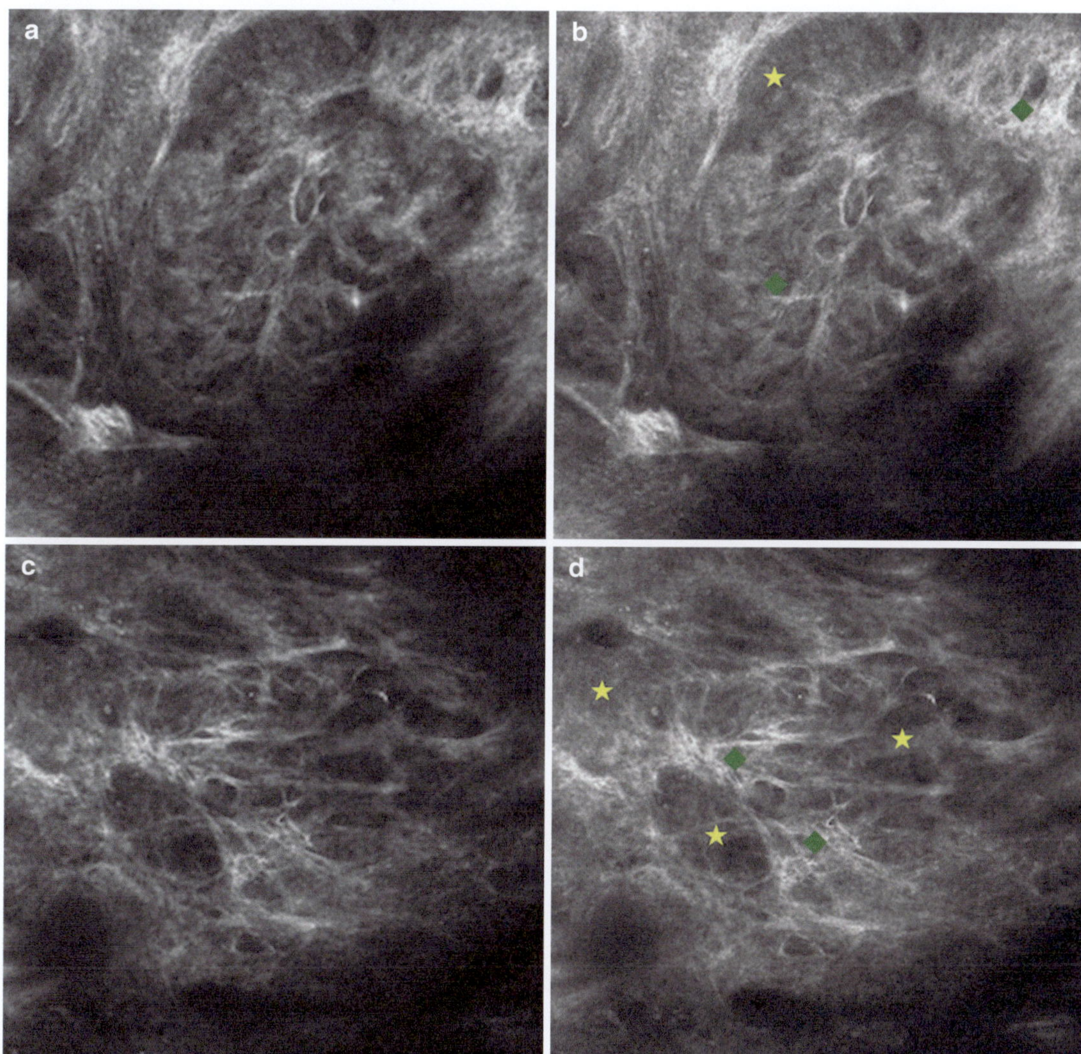

Fig. 6.11 IVCM features of sclerosing basal cell carcinoma (**a**–**d**)

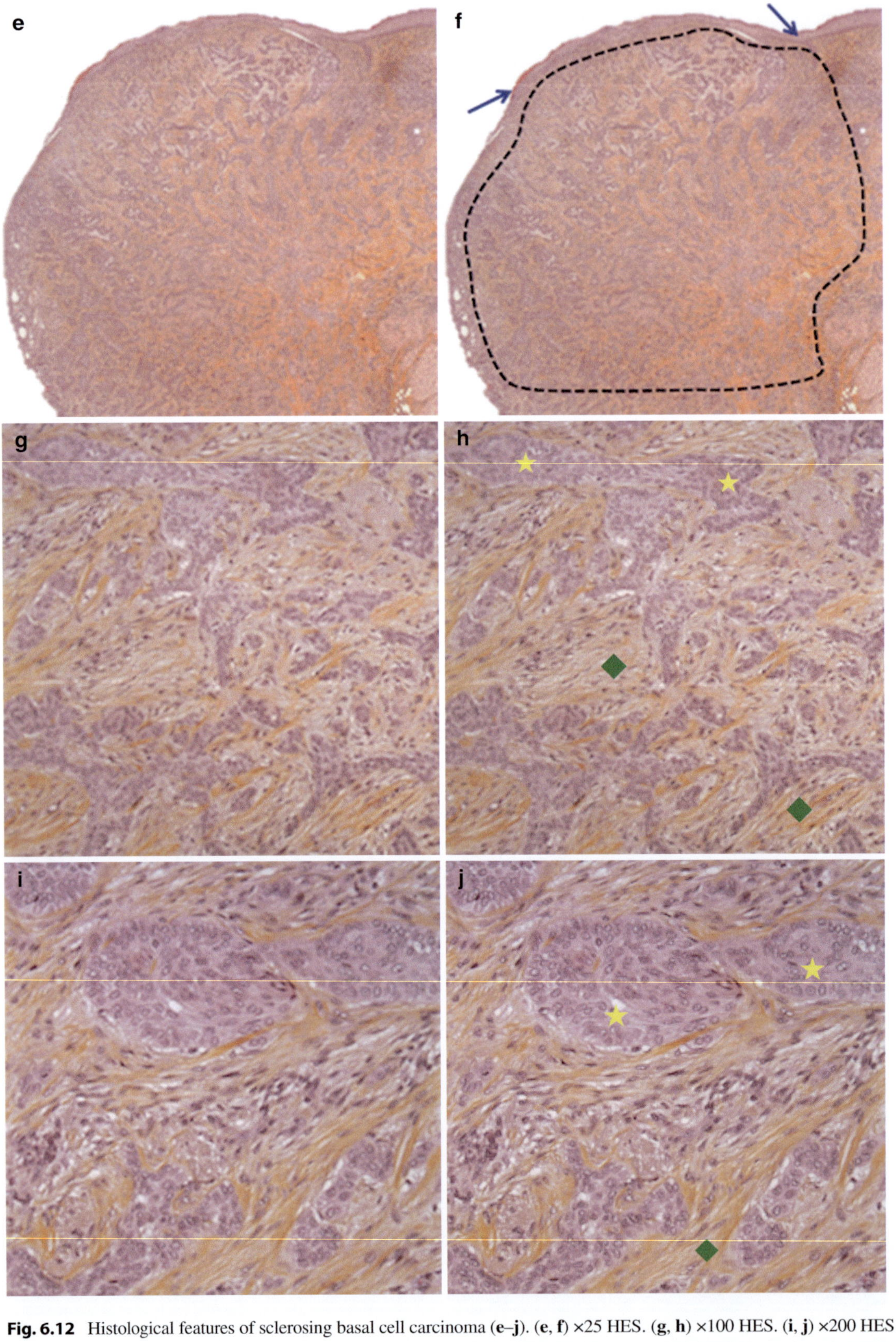

Fig. 6.12 Histological features of sclerosing basal cell carcinoma (**e–j**). (**e**, **f**) ×25 HES. (**g**, **h**) ×100 HES. (**i**, **j**) ×200 HES

References

1. Cinotti E, Singer A, Labeille B, Grivet D, Rubegni P, Douchet C, Cambazard F, Thuret G, Gain P, Perrot JL. Handheld in vivo reflectance confocal microscopy for the diagnosis of eyelid margin and conjunctival tumors. JAMA Ophthalmol. 2017;135(8):845–51. https://doi.org/10.1001/jamaophthalmol.2017.2019.
2. Cinotti E, Perrot JL, Campolmi N, Labeille B, Espinasse M, Grivet D, Thuret G, Gain P, Douchet C, Forest F, Haouas M, Cambazard F. The role of in vivo confocal microscopy in the diagnosis of eyelid margin tumors: 47 cases. J Am Acad Dermatol. 2014;71(5):912–918.e2. https://doi.org/10.1016/j.jaad.2014.05.060.

Part III

Melanocytic Lesions of the Eyelid

Benign Lesions with Basal Melanocyte Proliferation

7

Mathilde Kaspi, Thibaud Garcin, Cyril Habougit, Philippe Gain, Gilles Thuret, and Jean-Luc Perrot

Content

Abbreviations

Ab	Antibodies
HES	Hematoxylin-eosin-saffron stain
IVCM	In vivo reflectance confocal microscopy

M. Kaspi (✉) · T. Garcin · P. Gain · G. Thuret
Department of Ophthalmology, University Hospital of Saint-Etienne, Saint-Etienne Cedex 2, France
e-mail: mathilde.kaspi@gmail.com; garcinthibaud@gmail.com; philippe.gain@univ-st-etienne.fr; gilles.thuret@univ-st-etienne.fr

C. Habougit
Department of Pathology, University Hospital of Saint-Etienne, Saint-Etienne Cedex 2, France
e-mail: cyril.habougit@chu-st-etienne.fr

J.-L. Perrot
Department of Dermatology, University Hospital of Saint-Etienne, Saint-Etienne Cedex 2, France
e-mail: j.luc.perrot@chu-st-etienne.fr

7.1 Actinic Lentigo

Synonyms are solar lentigo and senile lentigo.

Actinic lentigo (Fig. 7.1) presents as a pigmented macule, with irregular contours, occurring on photo-exposed areas. The color is light brown and homogeneous. It can be single or multiple.

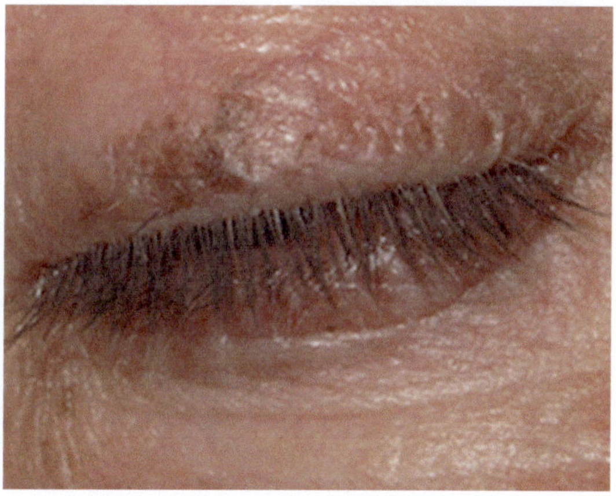

Fig. 7.1 Clinical aspect of actinic lentigo

© Springer Nature Switzerland AG 2020
M. Kaspi et al. (eds.), *Eyelid and Conjunctival Tumors*,
https://doi.org/10.1007/978-3-030-36606-3_7

The IVCM features are as follows (Fig. 7.2a–d):

- Normal supra-basal epidermis with regular honeycomb pattern (not shown here)
- Dermo-epidermal junction with increased density of elongated dermal papillae surrounded by a bright monomorphic layer of hyperreflective cells (cordlike rete ridges) (*orange arrows*) without atypical cells
- Absence of pagetoid cells

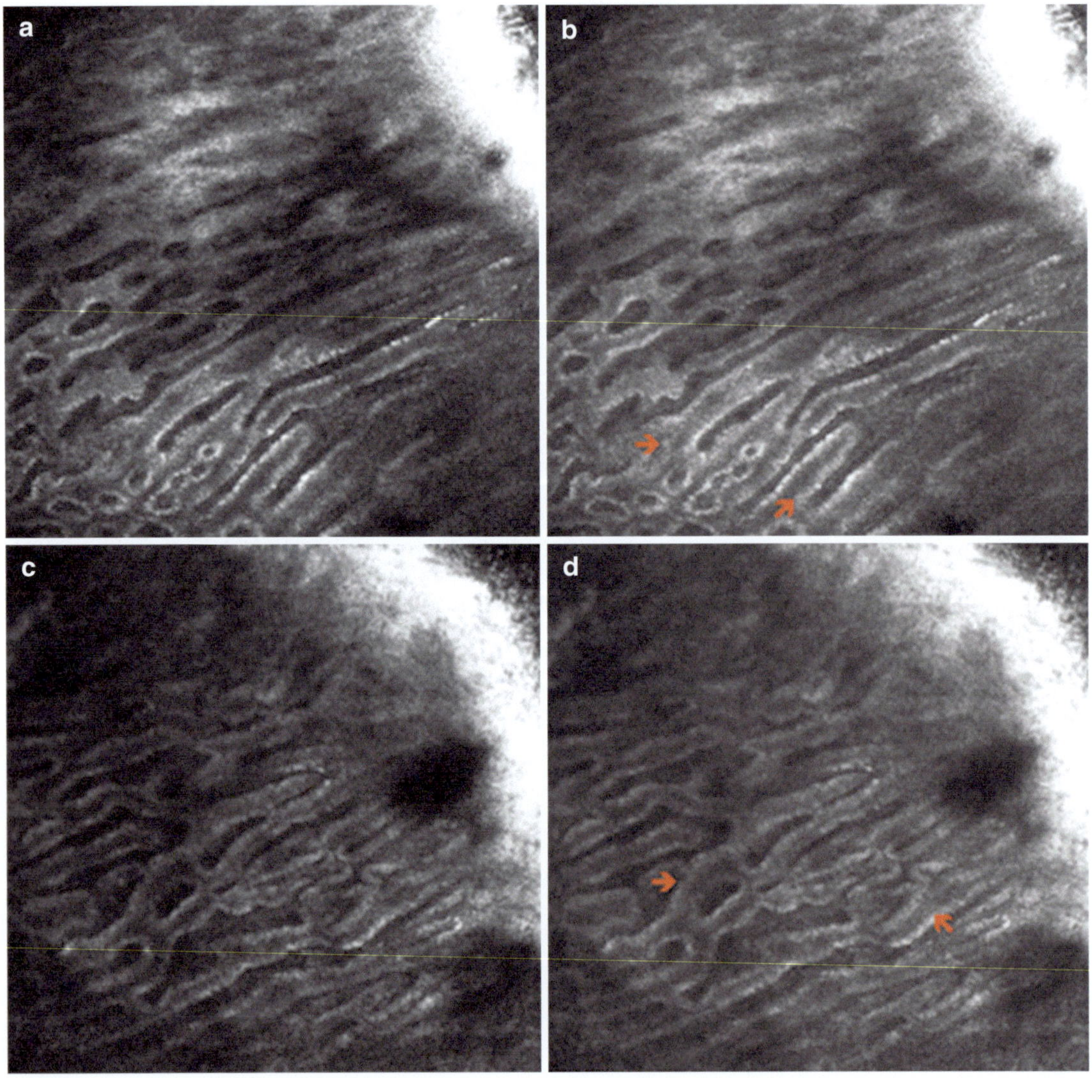

Fig. 7.2 IVCM features of actinic lentigo (**a**–**d**)

On optical microscopy the histologic features are as follows (Fig. 7.3e–h):

- At low magnification (e, f), the epidermis is organized into digitations (due to the lengthening of the epidermal ridges) and basal keratinocytes are hyperpigmented. Melanocytes can be slightly increased in number at the basal layer of the epidermis (*orange dotted lines*).
- At high magnification (g, h), melanocytes are regularly distributed at the basal layer of the epidermis without atypia or junctional nest. The epidermal ridges are hyperpigmented in places (*black arrows*).

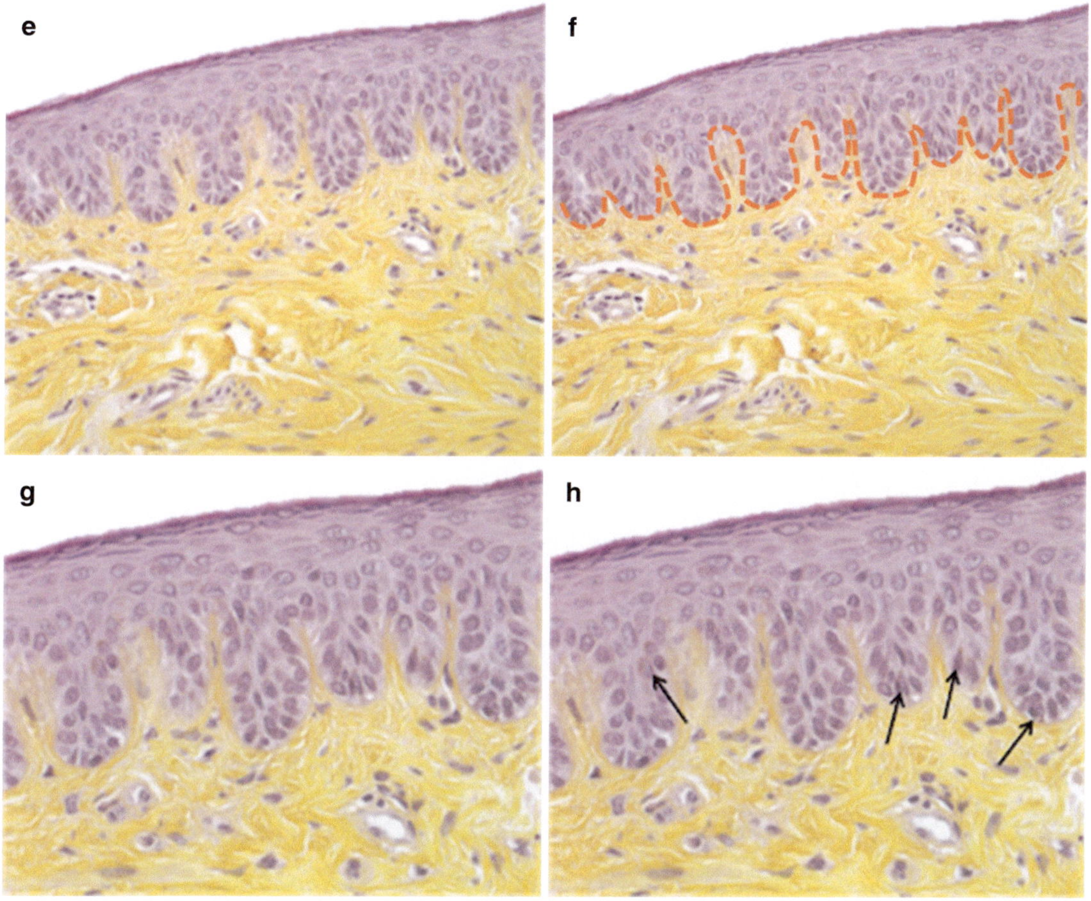

Fig. 7.3 Histological features of actinic lentigo (**e**–**h**). (**e**, **f**) ×100 HES. (**g**, **h**) ×400 HES

Benign Melanocytic Tumors

8

Mathilde Kaspi, Thibaud Garcin, Cyril Habougit,
Elisa Cinotti, Fabien Forest, and Jean-Luc Perrot

Contents

Abbreviations

HES Hematoxylin-eosin-saffron stain
IVCM In vivo reflectance confocal microscopy

Benign melanocytic lesions are represented by nevi. The clinical aspect of nevi is variable: pigmented or unpigmented, and flat or raised. They are classified into junctional, dermal, and compound according to the location of the melanocyte proliferation, respectively, purely intraepidermal, purely intradermal, and mixed (intraepidermal and intradermal).

M. Kaspi (✉) · T. Garcin
Department of Ophthalmology, University Hospital of Saint-Etienne, Saint-Etienne Cedex 2, France
e-mail: mathilde.kaspi@gmail.com; garcinthibaud@gmail.com

C. Habougit · F. Forest
Department of Pathology, University Hospital of Saint-Etienne, Saint-Etienne Cedex 2, France
e-mail: cyril.habougit@chu-st-etienne.fr; fabien.forest@chu-st-etienne.fr

E. Cinotti
Department of Dermatology, University of Siena, S. Maria alle Scotte Hospital, Siena, Italy
e-mail: elisa.cinotti@unisi.it

J.-L. Perrot
Department of Dermatology, University Hospital of Saint-Etienne, Saint-Etienne Cedex 2, France
e-mail: j.luc.perrot@chu-st-etienne.fr

© Springer Nature Switzerland AG 2020
M. Kaspi et al. (eds.), *Eyelid and Conjunctival Tumors*,
https://doi.org/10.1007/978-3-030-36606-3_8

8.1 Junctional Melanocytic Nevus

Nevi are generally junctional in childhood, and then evolve into compound and later dermal type. Junction activity decreases with age.

The clinical aspect (Fig. 8.1) of this junctional nevus is a brown macule of the free margin of the lower eyelid.

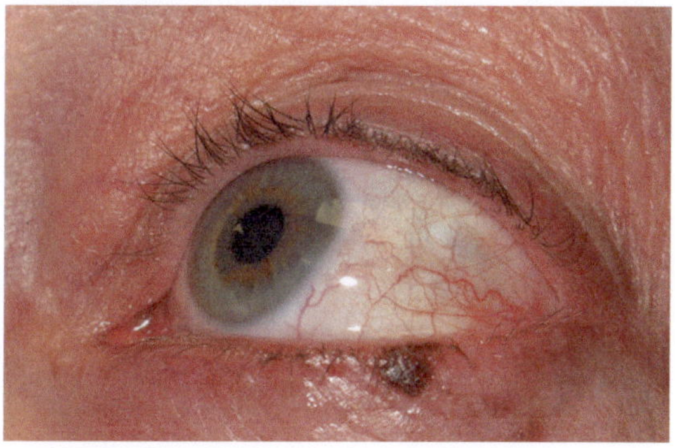

Fig. 8.1 Clinical aspect of junctional nevus

The IVCM features are as follows (Fig. 8.2a–d):

- Normal epidermis with regular honeycomb pattern (*red stars*)
- Round and regular hyperreflective homogeneous, roundish cells organized in nests at the dermo-epidermal junction (*yellow stars*) without atypical cells
- No pagetoid cells

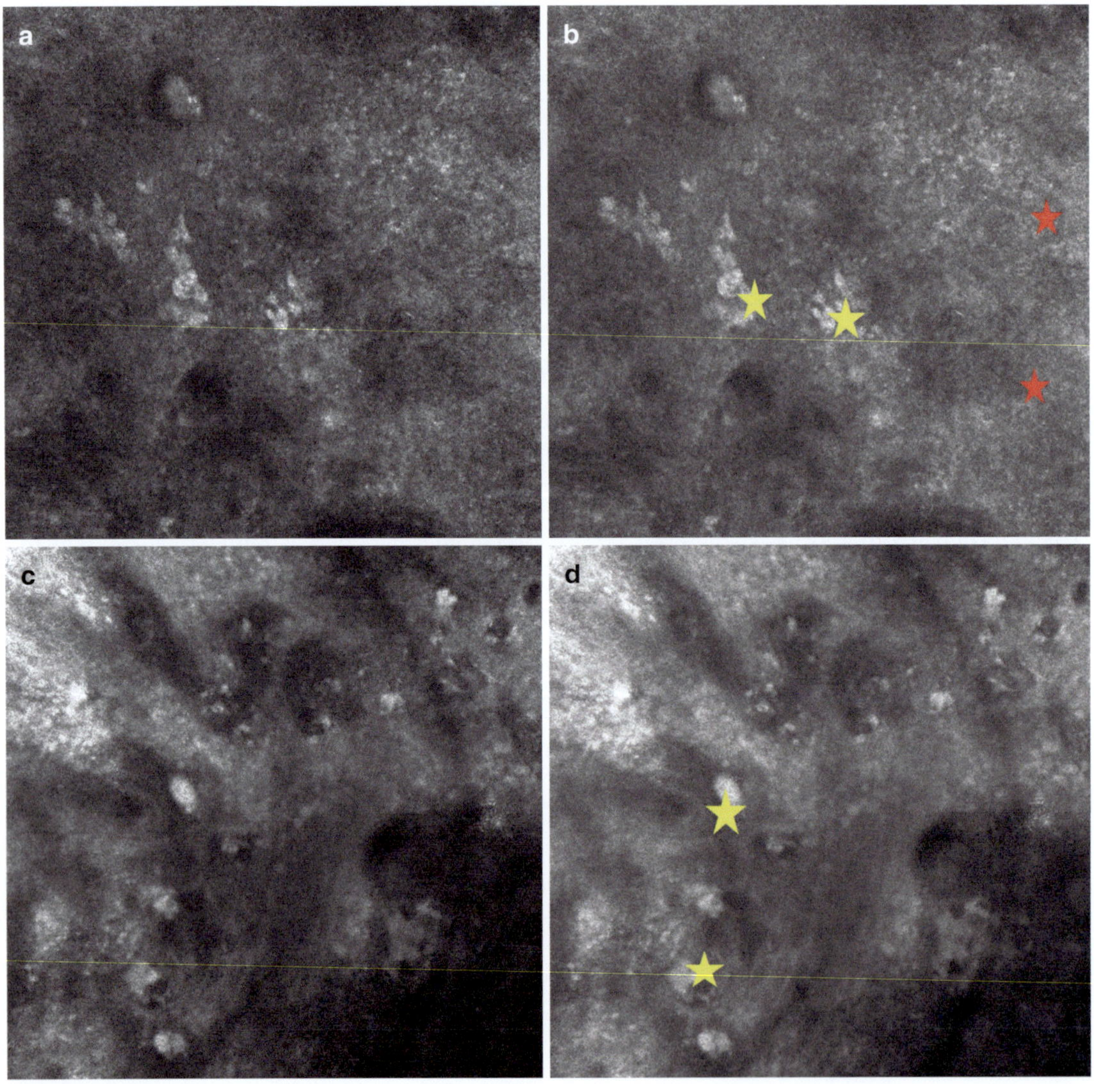

Fig. 8.2 IVCM features of junctional nevus (**a**–**d**)

On optical microscopy the histologic features are as follows (Fig. 8.3g–h):

- At low magnification (e, f), the lesion is composed of an exclusively intraepidermal melanocytic proliferation (*yellow stars*), above the basement membrane. There is no dermis component (*green diamonds*).
- At high magnification (g, h), melanocytes are arranged in nests (*blue stars*) at the tips of the rete ridges and have a lentiginous arrangement (*white circle*). The cells are small and epithelioid with pale and achromic cytoplasm.

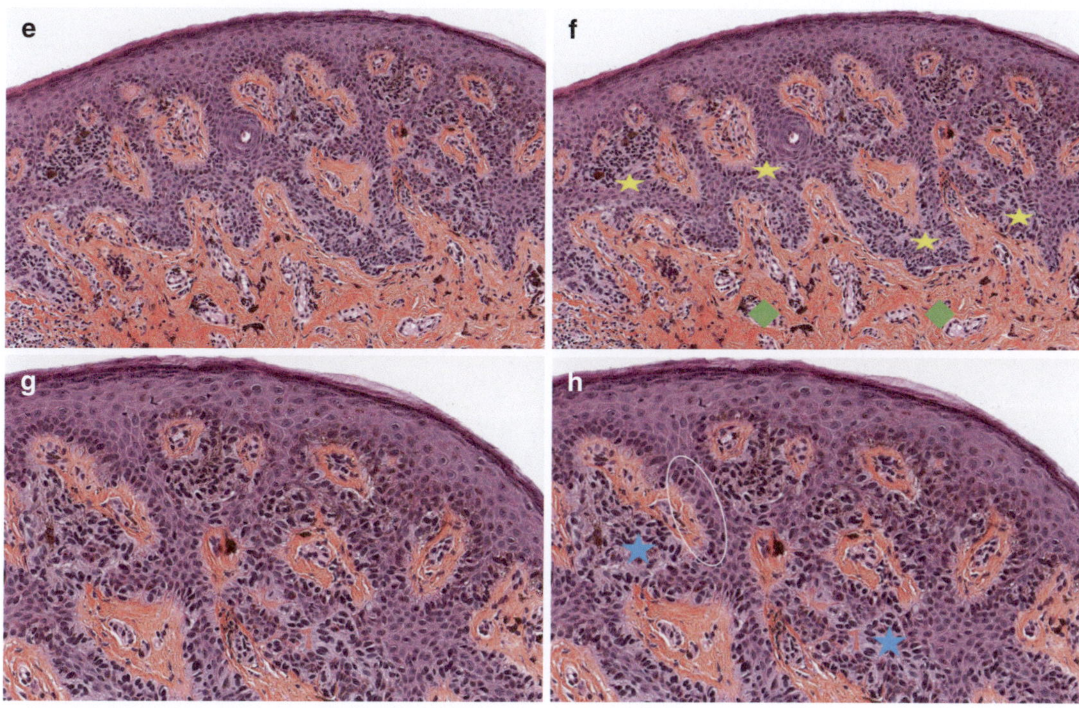

Fig. 8.3 Histological features of junctional nevus (**e–h**). (**e**, **f**) ×100 HES. (**g**, **h**) ×200 HES

8.2 Dermal Melanocytic Nevus

The clinical aspect (Fig. 8.4) of this dermal nevus is a well-limited brown homogeneous macule. Dermal nevi are often raised and achromic. They are the most frequent type of nevi of the eyelid.

The IVCM features are as follows (Fig. 8.5a–d):

- Normal epidermis with regular honeycomb pattern (*red stars*).
- Dermo-epidermal junction does not present any atypical cells.

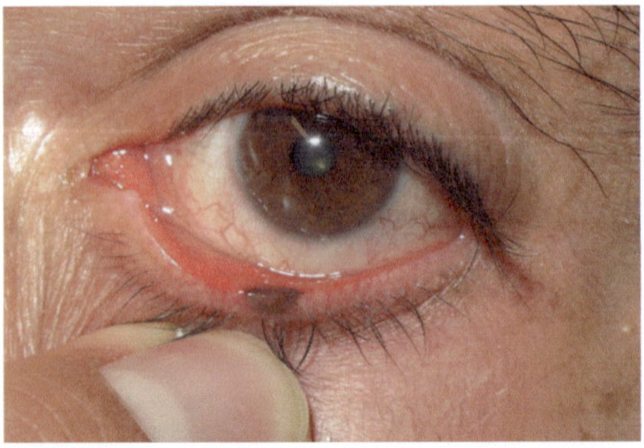

Fig. 8.4 Clinical aspect of dermal nevus

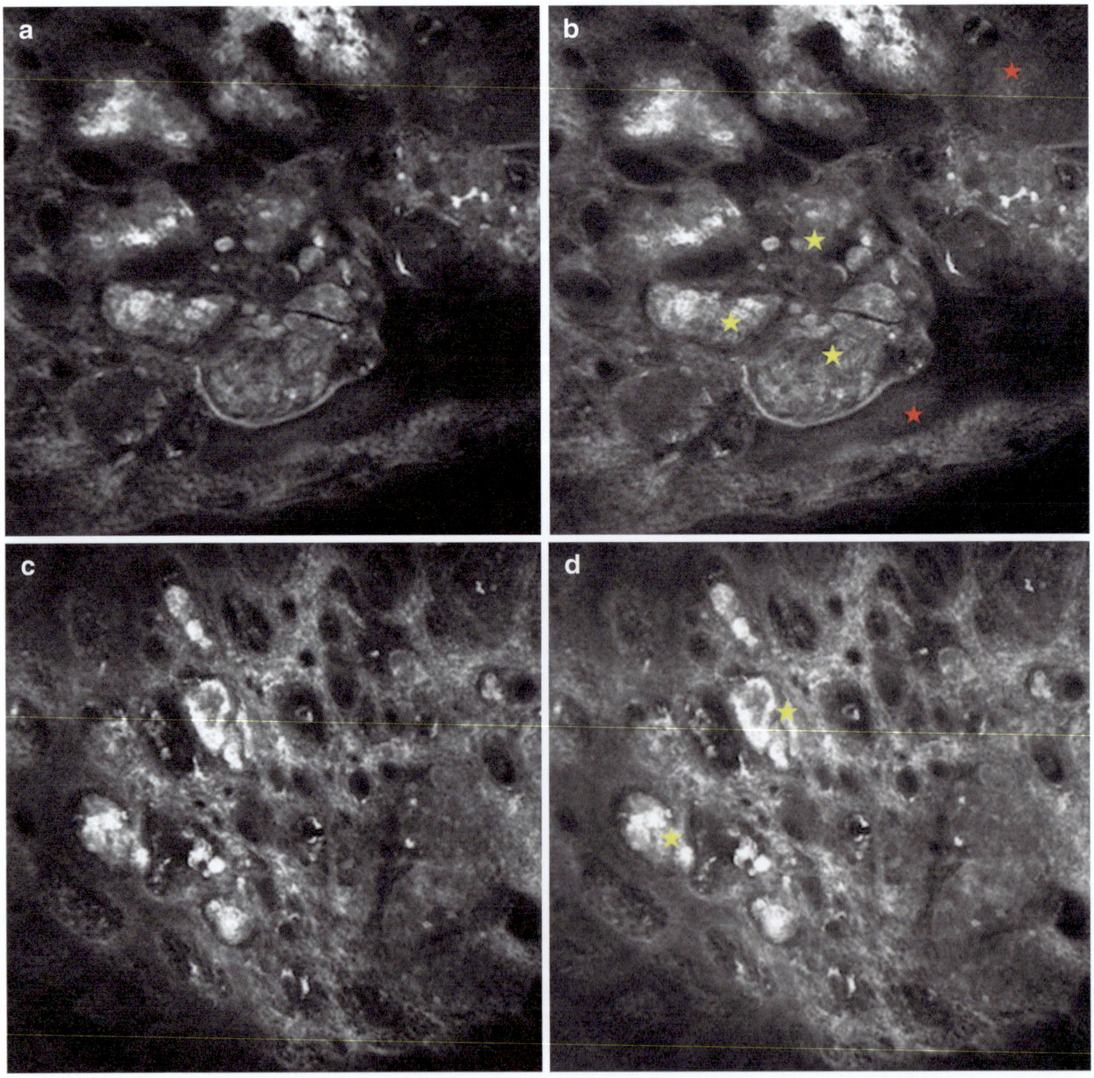

Fig. 8.5 IVCM features of dermal nevus (**a**–**d**)

- Hyperreflective, homogeneous, medium-sized (10–20 µm), roundish cells organized in nests (*yellow stars*) in the dermis.
- No pagetoid cells.

On optical microscopy the histologic features are as follows (Fig. 8.6e–h):

- At low magnification (e, f), the lesion is composed of a pure dermal melanocytic proliferation (*green dotted lines*), not connected with the epidermis.
- At high magnification (g, h), melanocytes are arranged in clusters (*green stars*), and nests (*yellow arrows*) in the dermis. The epidermis is not involved.

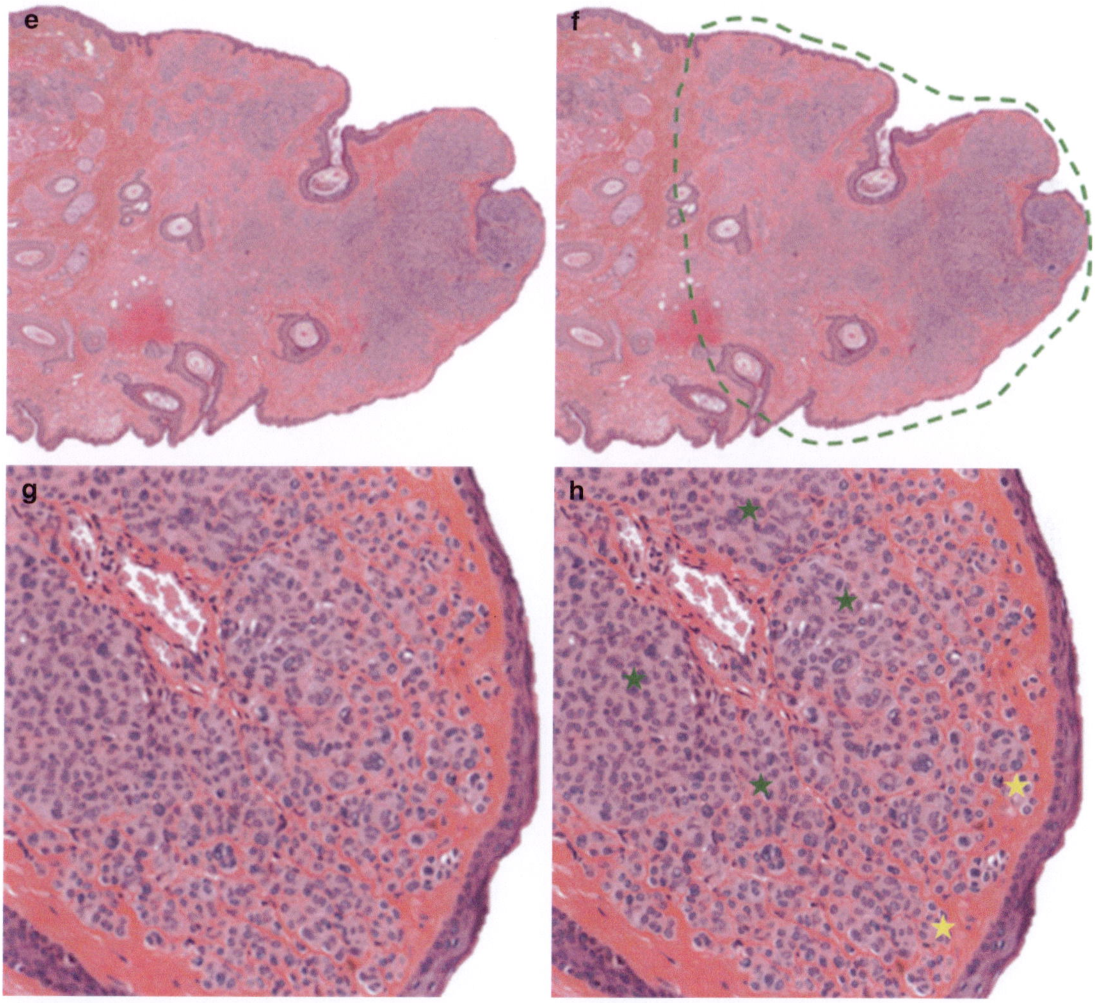

Fig. 8.6 Histological features of dermal nevus (**e**–**h**). (**e**, **f**) ×25 HES. (**g**, **h**) ×200 HES

8.3 Compound Melanocytic Nevus

The tarsal conjunctiva (Fig. 8.7) has a small macule, of homogeneous dark brown color, next to the tear point (*black arrow*).

Under IVCM compound nevus (Fig. 8.8a–d) has the features of both junctional and dermal nevus:

- Normal epidermis with regular honeycomb pattern, without disarrangement of the epithelial layers (not shown here)
- Dermo-epidermal junction (a, b) with large hyperreflective roundish and/or dendritic cells

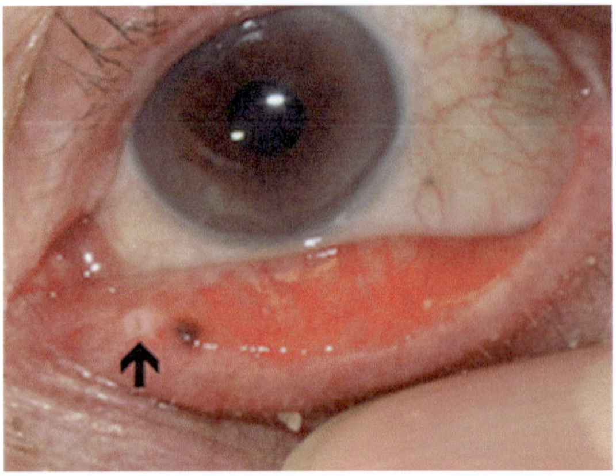

Fig. 8.7 Clinical aspect of compound nevus of the tarsal conjunctiva

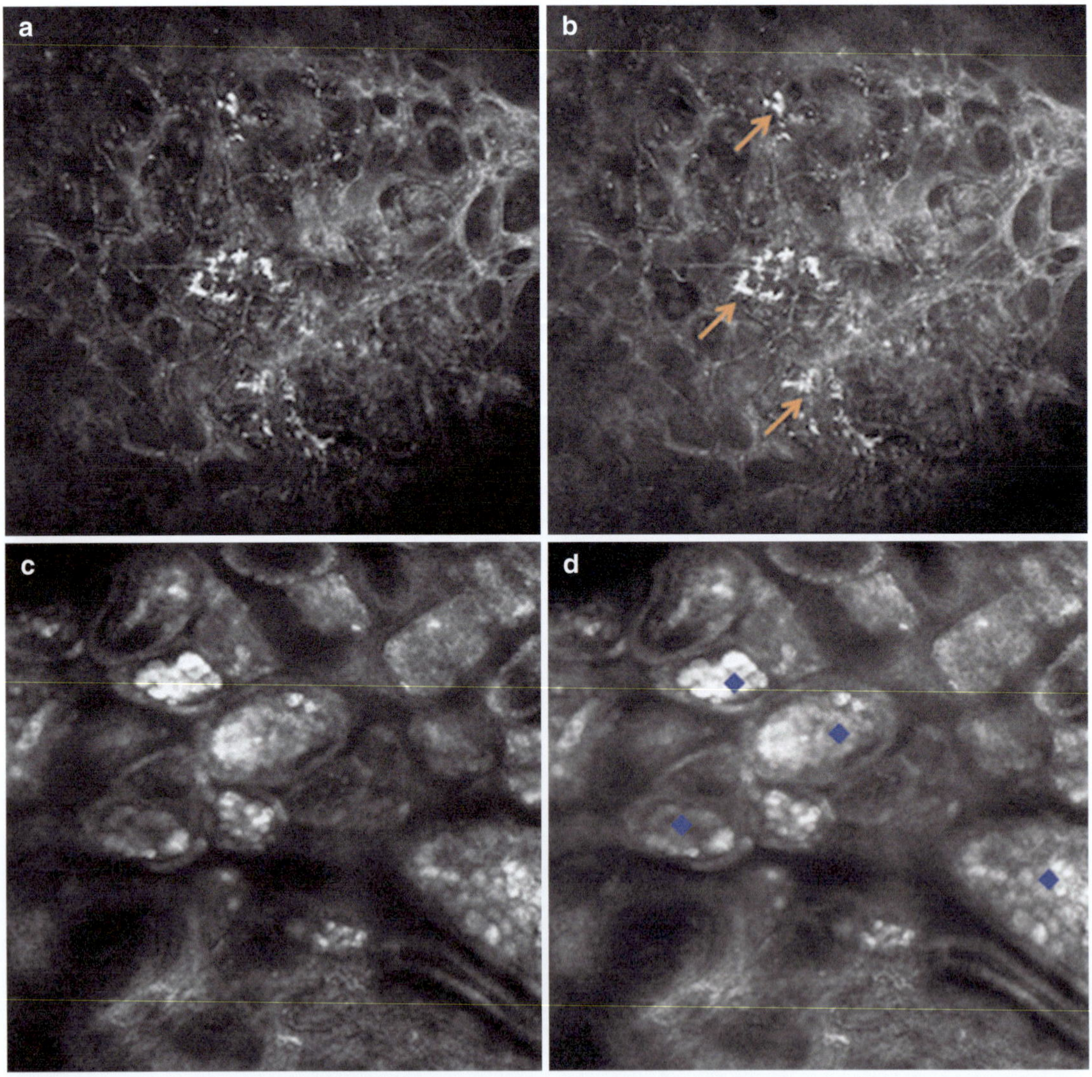

Fig. 8.8 IVCM features of compound nevus (**a**–**d**)

in single units and/or nests (*orange arrows*) corresponding to the junctional nevocytes
- Superficial dermis (c, d) with hyperreflective, homogeneous, medium-sized (10–20 μm), roundish cells organized in nests (*blue diamonds*)

On optical microscopy the histologic features are as follows (Fig. 8.9e–h):

- At low magnification (e, f), dermal melanocyte proliferation is organized in clusters (*blue diamonds*) in the superficial dermis, and in clusters (*green dotted lines*) in the deep dermis.
- At high magnification (g, h), the junctional melanocyte proliferation is rare and is arranged in micro-nests (*orange arrows*).

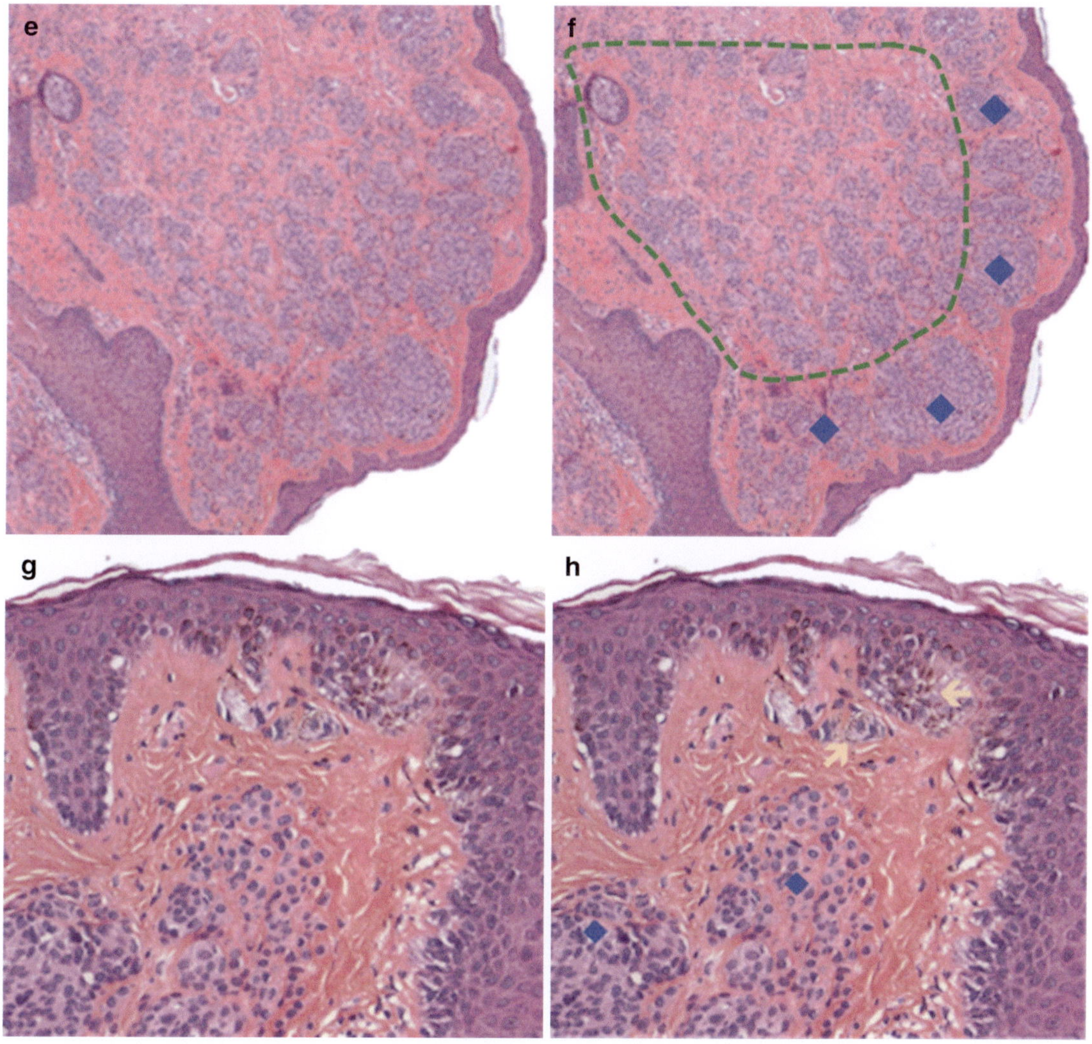

Fig. 8.9 Histological features of compound nevus (**e**–**h**). (**e**, **f**) ×50 HES. (**g**, **h**) ×200 HES

Malignant Melanocytic Tumors

9

Mathilde Kaspi, Thibaud Garcin, Cyril Habougit, Fabien Forest, Elisa Cinotti, and Jean-Luc Perrot

Contents

Abbreviations

Ab	Antibodies
HES	Hematoxylin-eosin-saffron stain
IVCM	In vivo reflectance confocal microscopy

M. Kaspi (✉) · T. Garcin
Department of Ophthalmology, University Hospital of Saint-Etienne, Saint-Etienne Cedex 2, France
e-mail: mathilde.kaspi@gmail.com; garcinthibaud@gmail.com

C. Habougit · F. Forest
Department of Pathology, University Hospital of Saint-Etienne, Saint-Etienne Cedex 2, France
e-mail: cyril.habougit@chu-st-etienne.fr; fabien.forest@chu-st-etienne.fr

E. Cinotti
Department of Dermatology, University of Siena, S. Maria alle Scotte Hospital, Siena, Italy
e-mail: elisa.cinotti@unisi.it

J.-L. Perrot
Department of Dermatology, University Hospital of Saint-Etienne, Saint-Etienne Cedex 2, France
e-mail: j.luc.perrot@chu-st-etienne.fr

© Springer Nature Switzerland AG 2020
M. Kaspi et al. (eds.), *Eyelid and Conjunctival Tumors*,
https://doi.org/10.1007/978-3-030-36606-3_9

9.1 Lentigo Maligna

Lentigo maligna occurs in photo-exposed areas. Atypical melanocytes proliferate along the basement membrane without crossing it: lentigo maligna is a melanoma in situ. When melanocytes cross the basement membrane and invade the dermis the tumor is called lentigo maligna melanoma.

Clinically, lentigo maligna (Fig. 9.1) presents as a nonhomogeneous pigmented macule on sun-exposed skin, with irregular contours.

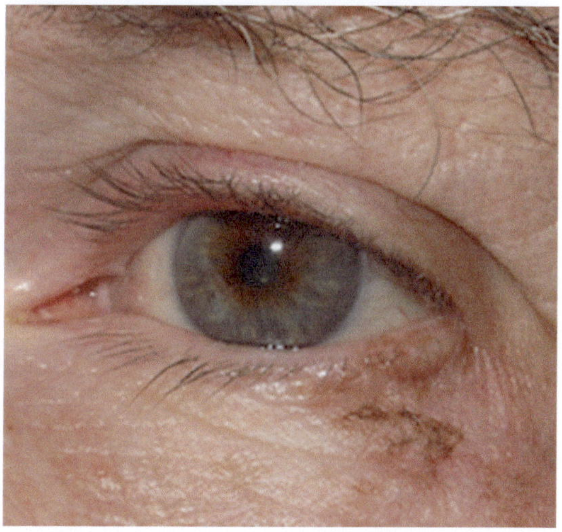

Fig. 9.1 Clinical aspect of actinic lentigo

The IVCM features are as follows (Fig. 9.2a–d):

- Relatively well-preserved epidermis with regular honeycomb pattern (not shown here)
- Atypical roundish and/or dendritic cells (that correspond to large cells of different shapes and sizes) at the dermo-epidermal junction (*orange stars*) and the suprabasal layers of the epidermis (pagetoid cells*; blue arrows*)

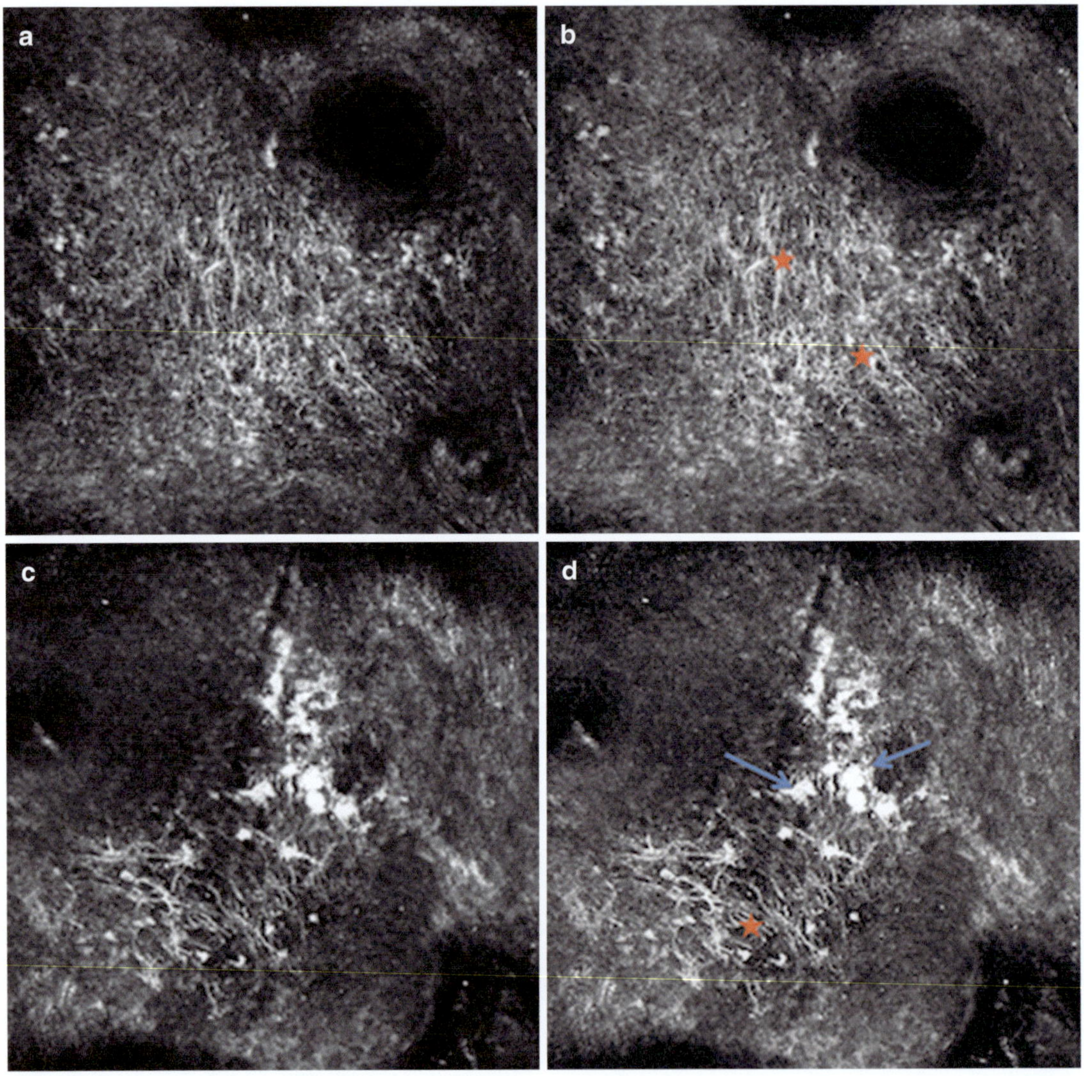

Fig. 9.2 IVCM features of actinic lentigo (**a**–**d**)

On optical microscopy the histologic features are as follows (Fig. 9.3e–i):

– At low magnification (e, f), melanocytic proliferation (*red dotted line*) occurs along the basement membrane, without crossing it.
– Melanocytes are marked in red in immunohistochemistry by the anti-Melan-A antibody (g).
– At high magnification (h, i), atypical melanocytes proliferate along the basement membrane in a lentiginous mode (*black circle*). Some nests at the level of the basement membrane are visible (*blue arrows*).

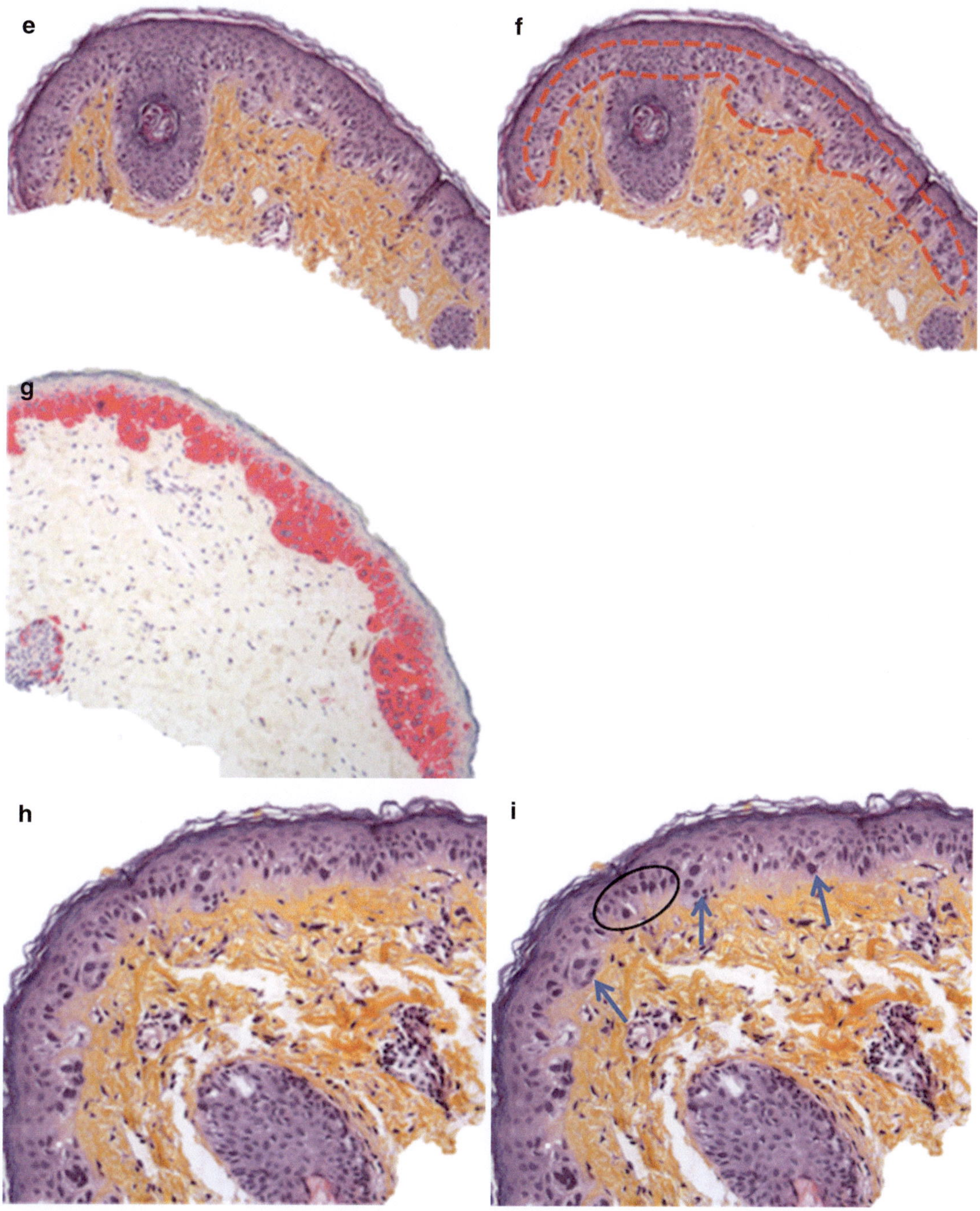

Fig. 9.3 Histological features of actinic lentigo (**c–i**). (**e, f**) ×100 HES. (**g**) ×100 Anti-Melan-A Ab. (**h, i**) ×200 HES

9.2 Melanoma

Eyelid melanomas represent less than 1% of palpebral malignant tumors. In melanoma, atypical melanocytes are present in the epidermis and dermis. The most frequent histological types of palpebral melanomas are:

- Superficial spreading melanoma (SMM)
- Lentigo malignant melanoma (LMM)

The clinical aspect (Fig. 9.4) of this eyelid melanoma is a heterogeneous and irregular dark brown pigmentation.

The IVCM features are as follows (Fig. 9.5a–e):

- Disarranged epithelium (a–c) with large hyperreflective dendritic (*red circle*) and roundish pagetoid cells (*yellow arrows* and *image c*)
- Large hyperreflective polymorphic cells (*orange stars*) in the superficial dermis (d, e) in case of invasive melanoma

On optical microscopy the histologic features are as follows (Fig. 9.6f–k):

- At low magnification (f–i), melanocytic proliferation invades the dermis (*black circle*), and its intraepidermal lateral component looks lentiginous (*blue dotted lines*). Melanocytes are stained in red by anti-Melan-A antibody.
- At high magnification (j, k), the dermal component is composed of melanocytes arranged in nests (*green diamonds*). The intraepidermal lateral component is lentiginous (*blue dotted line*). Some mitoses are visible (*black arrows*).

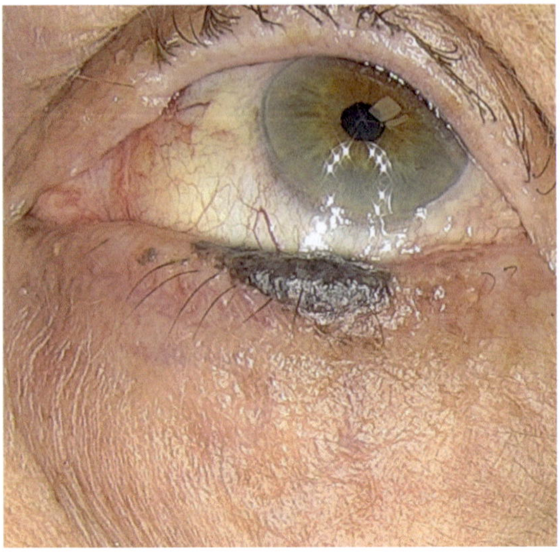

Fig. 9.4 Clinical aspect of eyelid melanoma

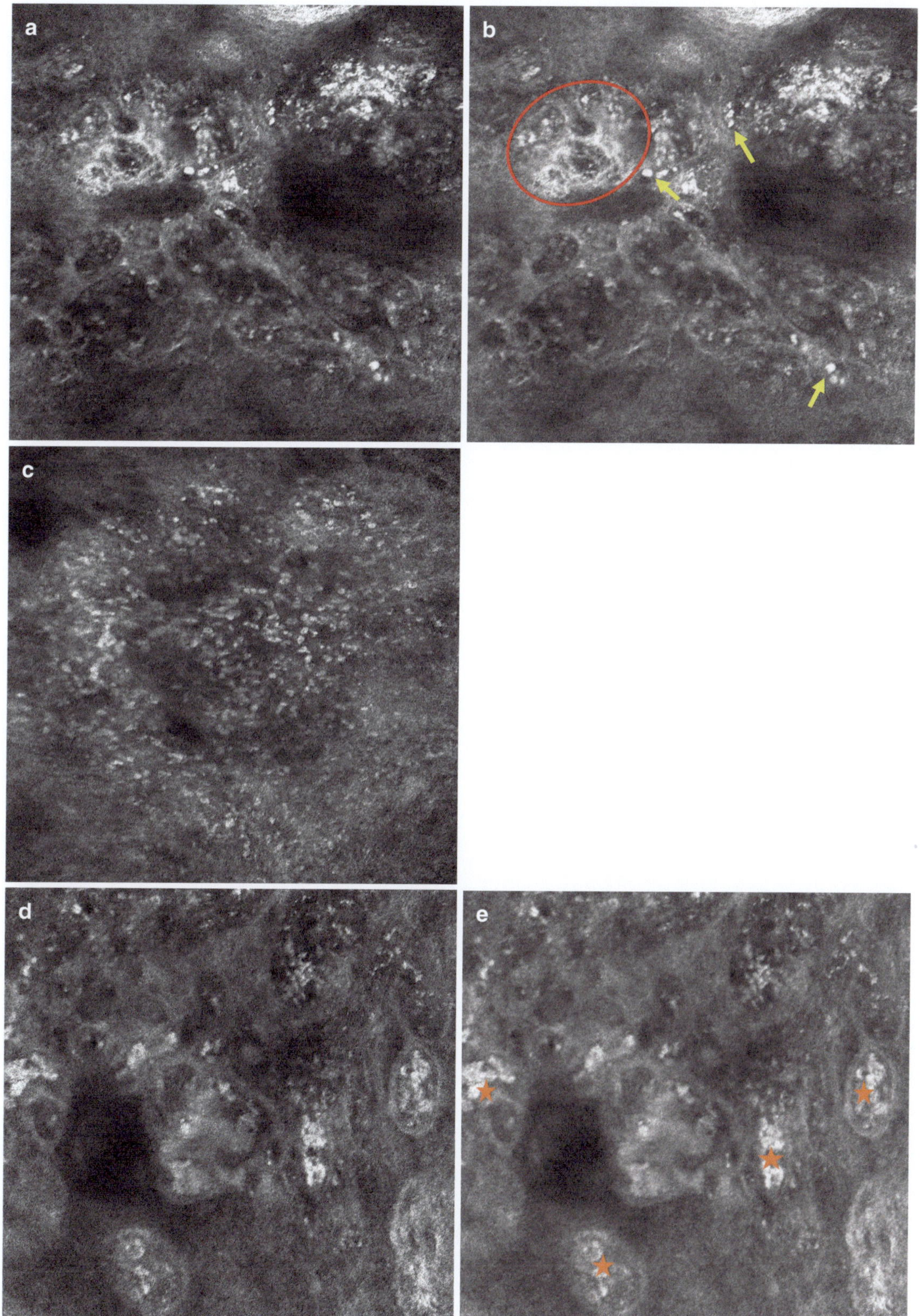

Fig. 9.5 IVCM features of eyelid melanoma (**a–e**)

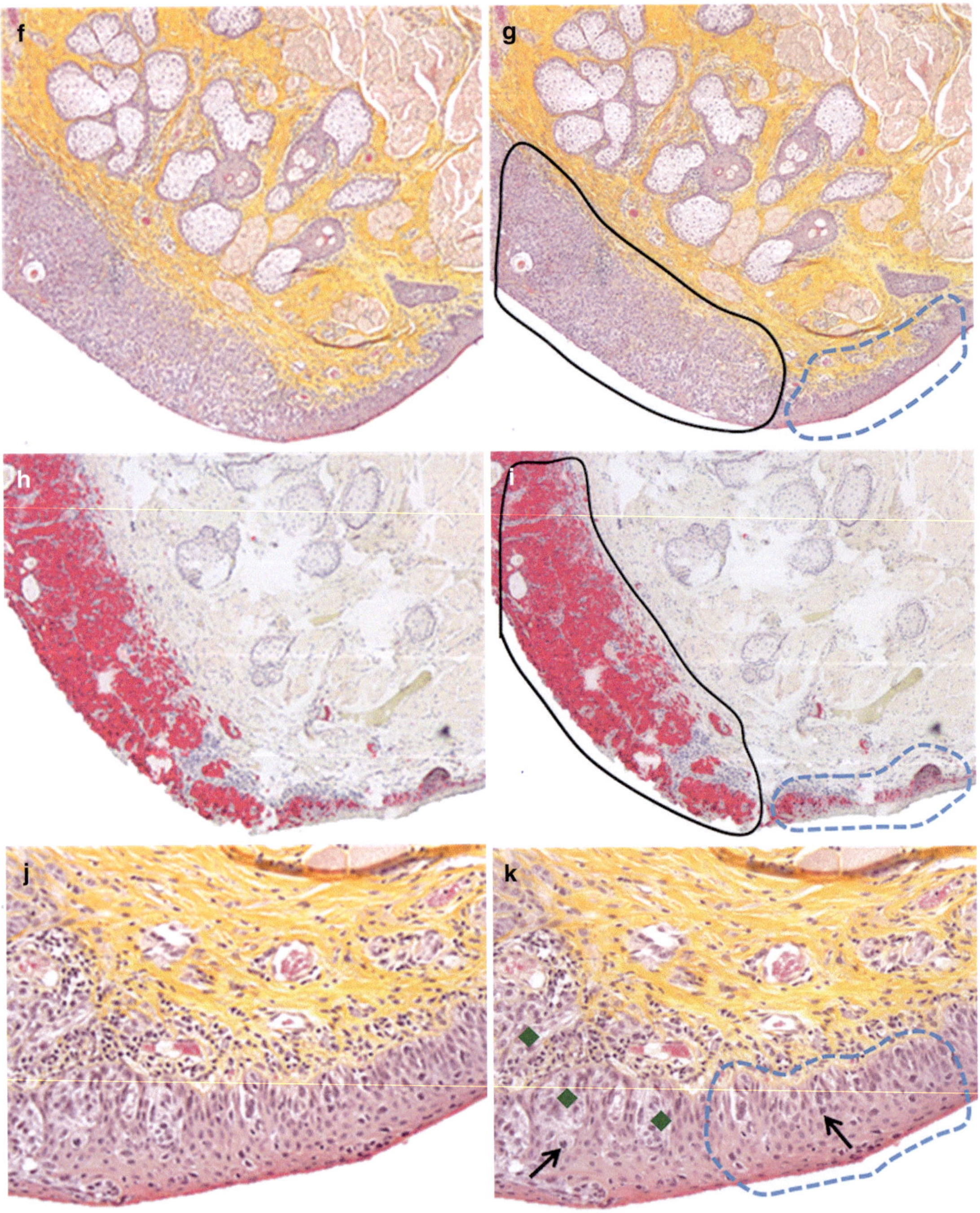

Fig. 9.6 Histological features of eyelid melanoma (**f**–**k**). (**f**, **g**) ×50 HES. (**h**, **i**) ×50 Anti-Melan-A Ab. (**j**, **k**) ×200 HES

Part IV

Non-epidermal and Non-melanocytic Lesions of the Eyelid

Appendageal Tumors 10

Mathilde Kaspi, Thibaud Garcin, Elisa Cinotti,
Damien Grivet, Cyril Habougit,
and Jean-Luc Perrot

Contents

Abbreviations

HES Hematoxylin-eosin-saffron stain
IVCM In vivo reflectance confocal microscopy

M. Kaspi (✉) · T. Garcin · D. Grivet
Department of Ophthalmology, University Hospital of Saint-Etienne, Saint-Etienne Cedex 2, France
e-mail: mathilde.kaspi@gmail.com; garcinthibaud@gmail.com; damien.grivet@chu-st-etienne.fr

E. Cinotti
Department of Dermatology, University of Siena, S. Maria alle Scotte Hospital, Siena, Italy
e-mail: elisa.cinotti@unisi.it

C. Habougit
Department of Pathology, University Hospital of Saint-Etienne, Saint-Etienne Cedex 2, France
e-mail: cyril.habougit@chu-st-etienne.fr

J.-L. Perrot
Department of Dermatology, University Hospital of Saint-Etienne, Saint-Etienne Cedex 2, France
e-mail: j.luc.perrot@chu-st-etienne.fr

© Springer Nature Switzerland AG 2020
M. Kaspi et al. (eds.), *Eyelid and Conjunctival Tumors*,
https://doi.org/10.1007/978-3-030-36606-3_10

10.1 Benign Appendageal Tumors

10.1.1 Trichoepithelioma

Trichoepithelioma is a benign appendageal tumor of pilar origin.

The clinical aspect (Fig. 10.1) of trichoepithelioma is a white or flesh-colored smooth-surface pearly papule or nodule that may include telangiectasia. It may be often clinically mistaken for basal cell carcinoma.

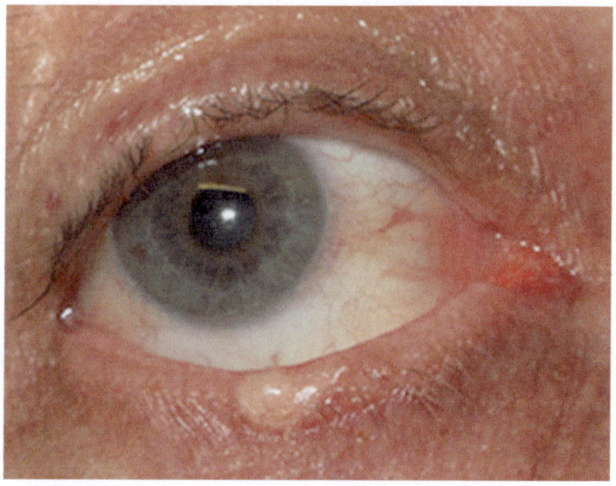

Fig. 10.1 Clinical aspect of trichoepithelioma

The IVCM features are as follows (Fig. 10.2a–d):

- Epidermis with regular honeycomb pattern (not shown here).
- Superficial dermis with low and medium reflective roundish and branching islands of uniform basaloid cells (*yellow stars*) in a hyperreflective abundant stroma, associated with hyperreflective small keratinous pseudocysts (*orange arrows*) and epithelial structures resembling hair papillae or abortive hair follicles (*blue diamond*).
- Focal connection of tumor islands to the epidermis and peripheral palisading are possible findings.

The differential diagnosis with basal cell carcinoma is challenging.

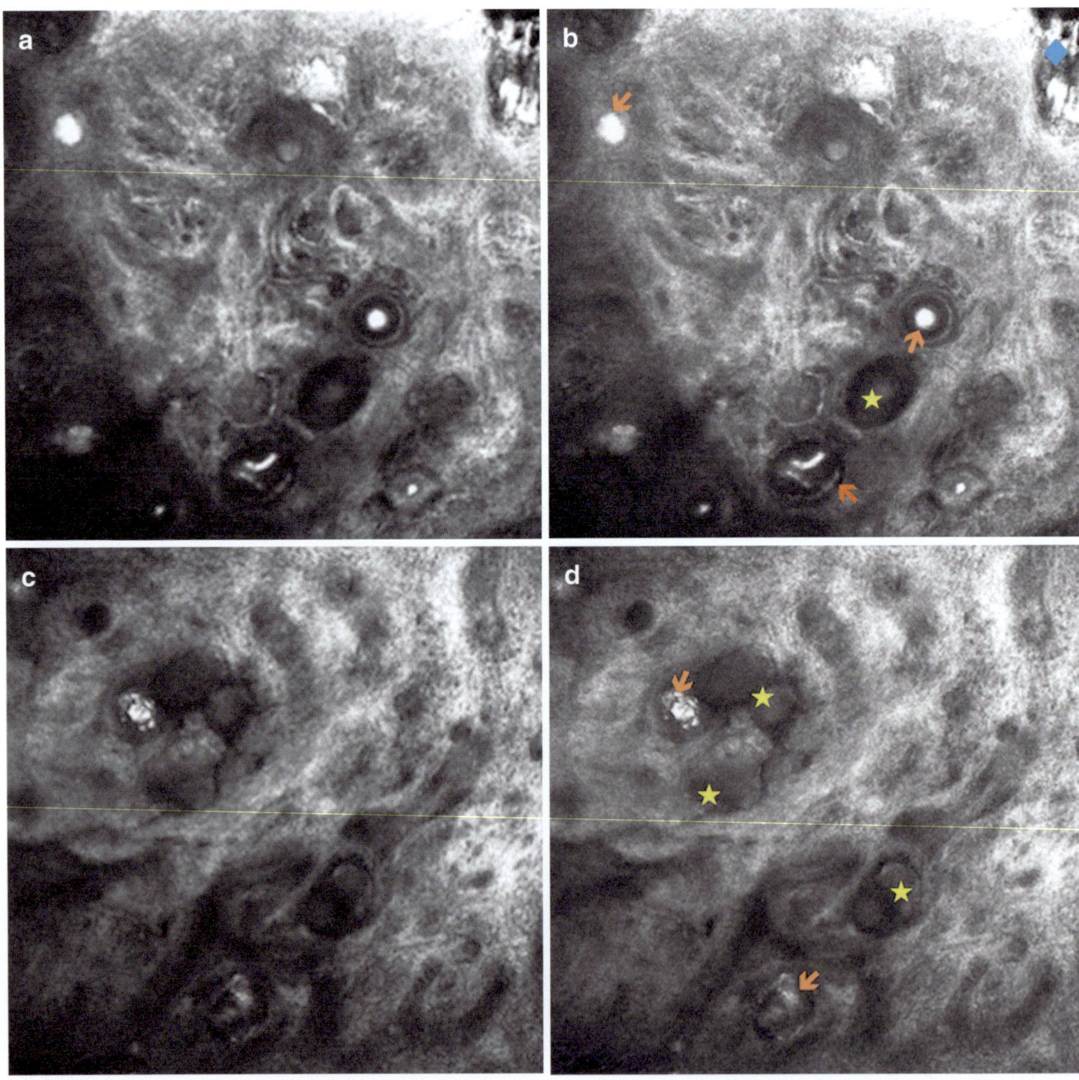

Fig. 10.2 IVCM features of trichoepithelioma (**a**–**d**)

On optical microscopy the histologic features are as follows (Fig. 10.3e–h):

- At low magnification (e, f), the lesion consists of an intradermal proliferation of uniform basaloid cell islands that form cords (*yellow stars*).
- At high magnification (g, h), these cellular cords have a trabecular organization (*yellow stars*) and contain keratinous pseudocysts (*orange arrows*). The stroma is prominent and loosely arranged.

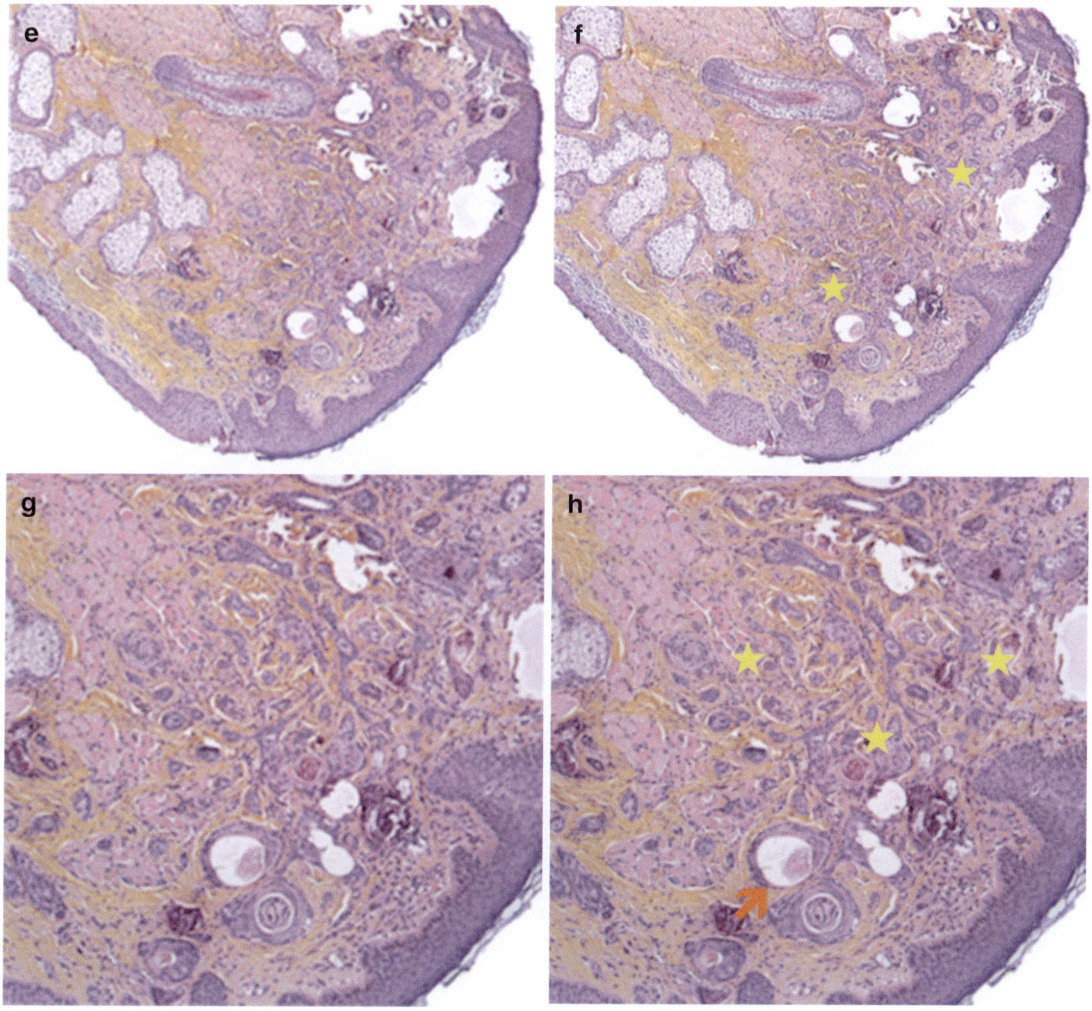

Fig. 10.3 Histological features of trichoepithelioma (**e**–**h**). (**e**, **f**) ×25 HES. (**g**, **h**) ×100 HES

10.1.2 Hidrocystoma

Hidrocystoma is a retention cyst of eccrine or apocrine sebaceous glands.

The clinical aspect (Fig. 10.4) of hidrocystoma is a translucent or pigmented cyst whose content may be serous, gelatinous, or hemorrhagic.

The IVCM features are as follows (Fig. 10.5a–d):

- Normal epidermis with regular honeycomb pattern (*red stars*)
- Dermo-epidermal junction that is not easily identifiable (*orange arrows*)

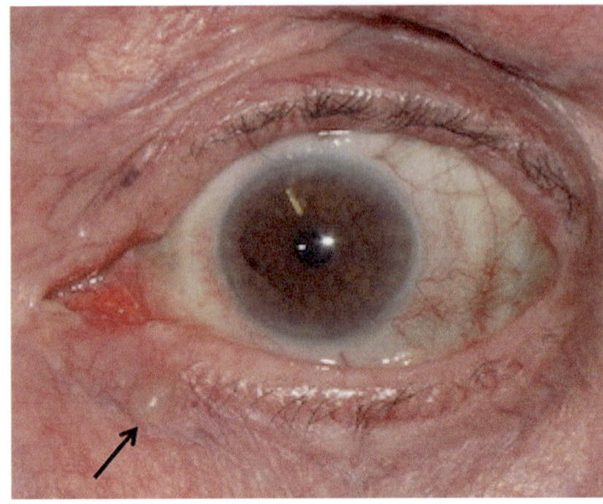

Fig. 10.4 Clinical aspect of hidrocystoma

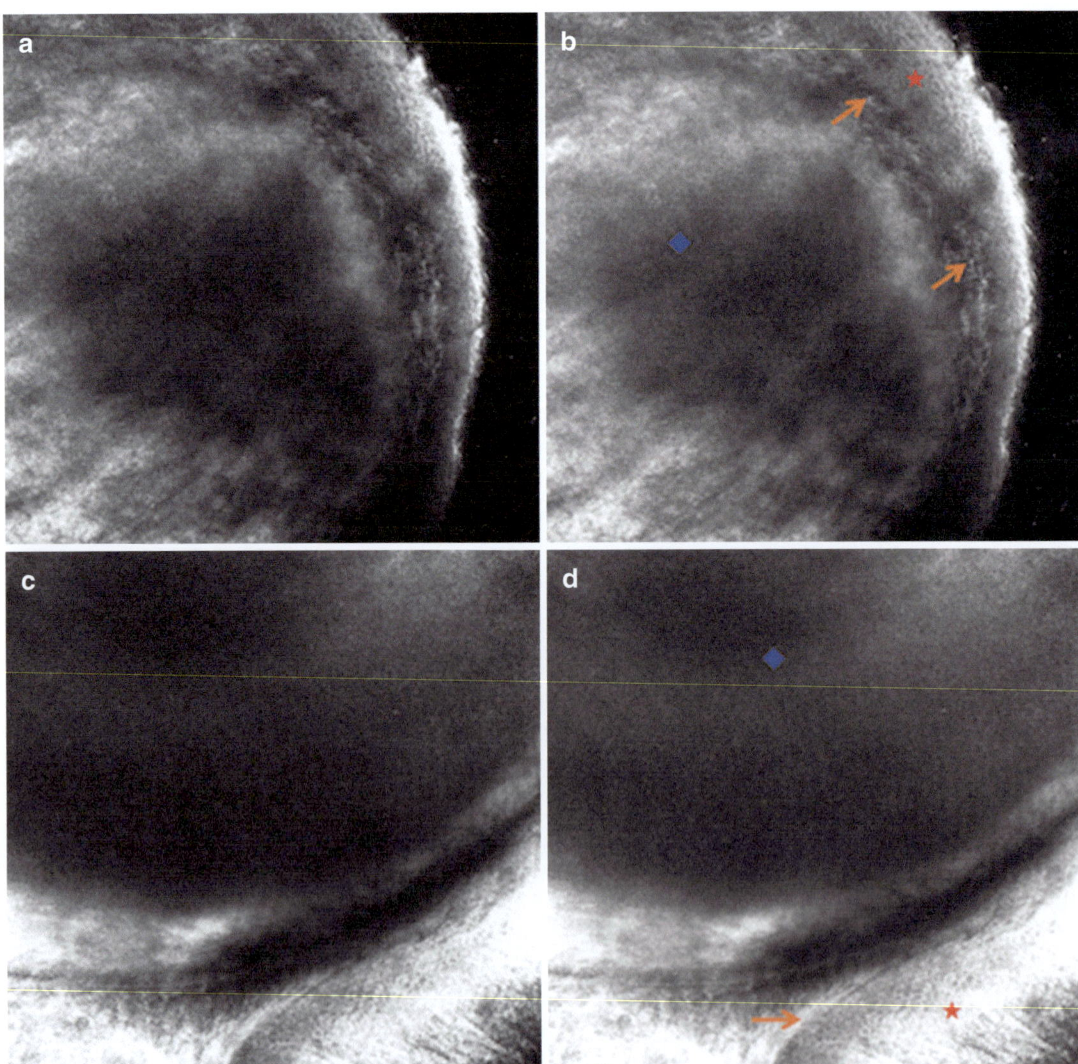

Fig. 10.5 IVCM features of hidrocystoma (**a**–**d**)

- Cyst located in the dermis, optically nonreflective, homogeneous (*blue diamonds*), and well limited by an epithelium

On optical microscopy the histologic features are as follows (Fig. 10.6e–h):

- At low magnification (e, f), the cyst lumen contains foamy elements (*blue diamonds*).
- At high magnification (g, h), the endoluminal base of the cyst is bordered by cubic epithelial cells (*green arrows*). Myoepithelial cells are present (*black arrows*).

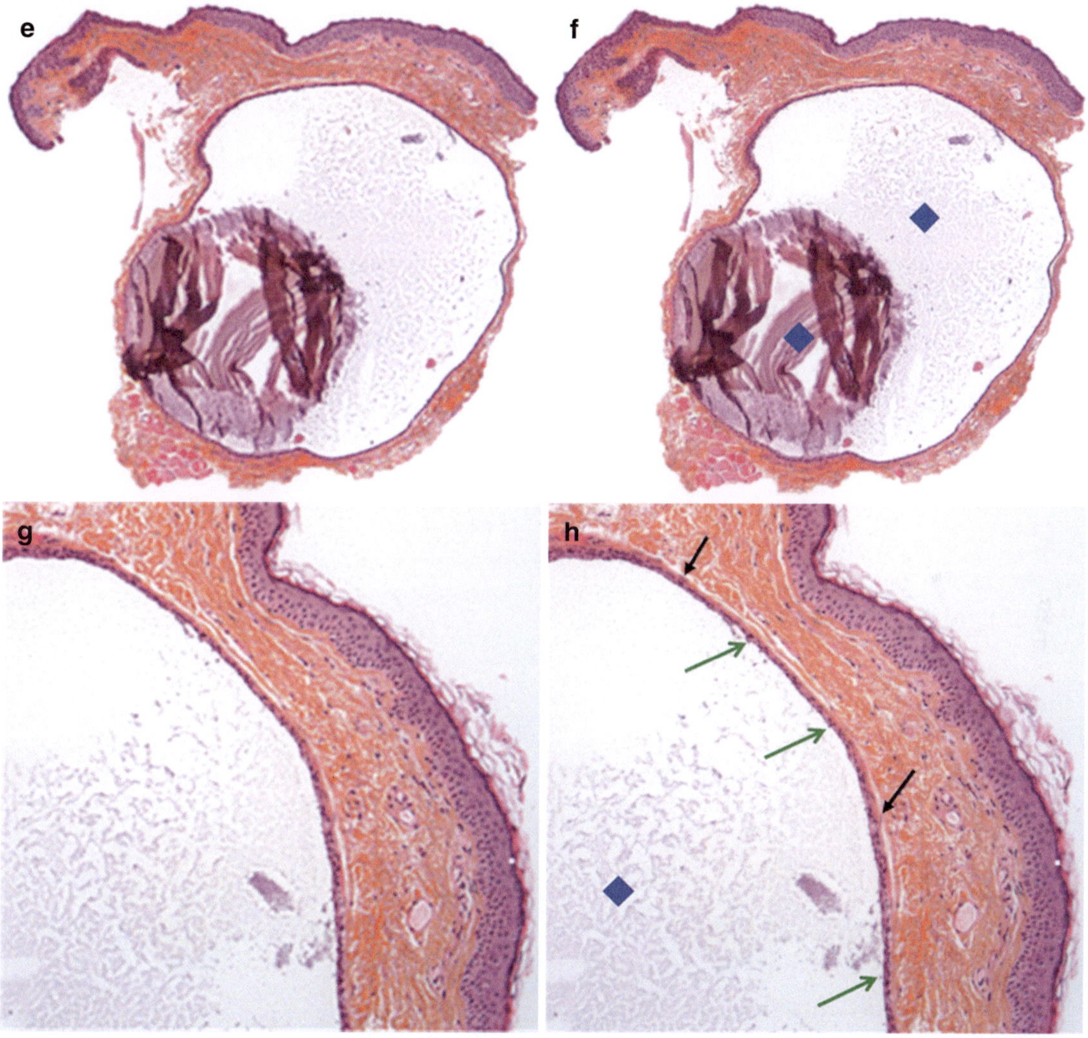

Fig. 10.6 Histological features of hidrocystoma (**e**–**h**). (**e**–**j**) ×50 HES. (**g**, **h**) ×100 HES

10.1.3 Syringoma

Syringoma is a benign appendageal tumor of the eccrine glands.

Syringoma (Fig. 10.7) is usually found as multiple small papules on the lower eyelids and cheeks, white or yellow in color.

The IVCM features are as follows (Fig. 10.8a–d):

- Normal epidermis is seen (not shown here).
- Superficial dermis is seen with ductal structures visible as hyporeflective lacunae (*yellow stars*) with some hyperreflective material inside; solid nests and strands of cells (*green diamonds*) are also present.

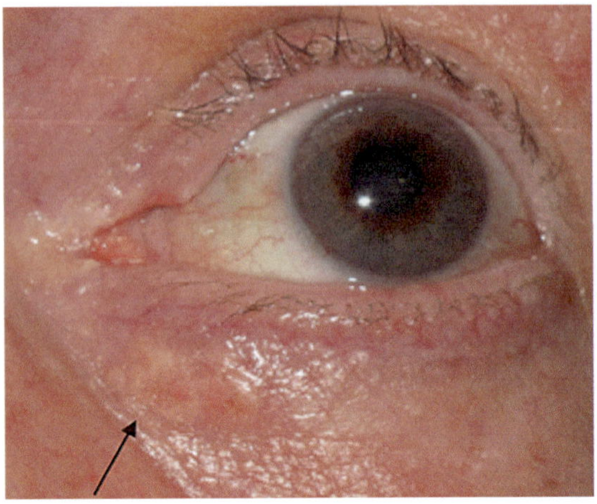

Fig. 10.7 Clinical aspect of syringoma

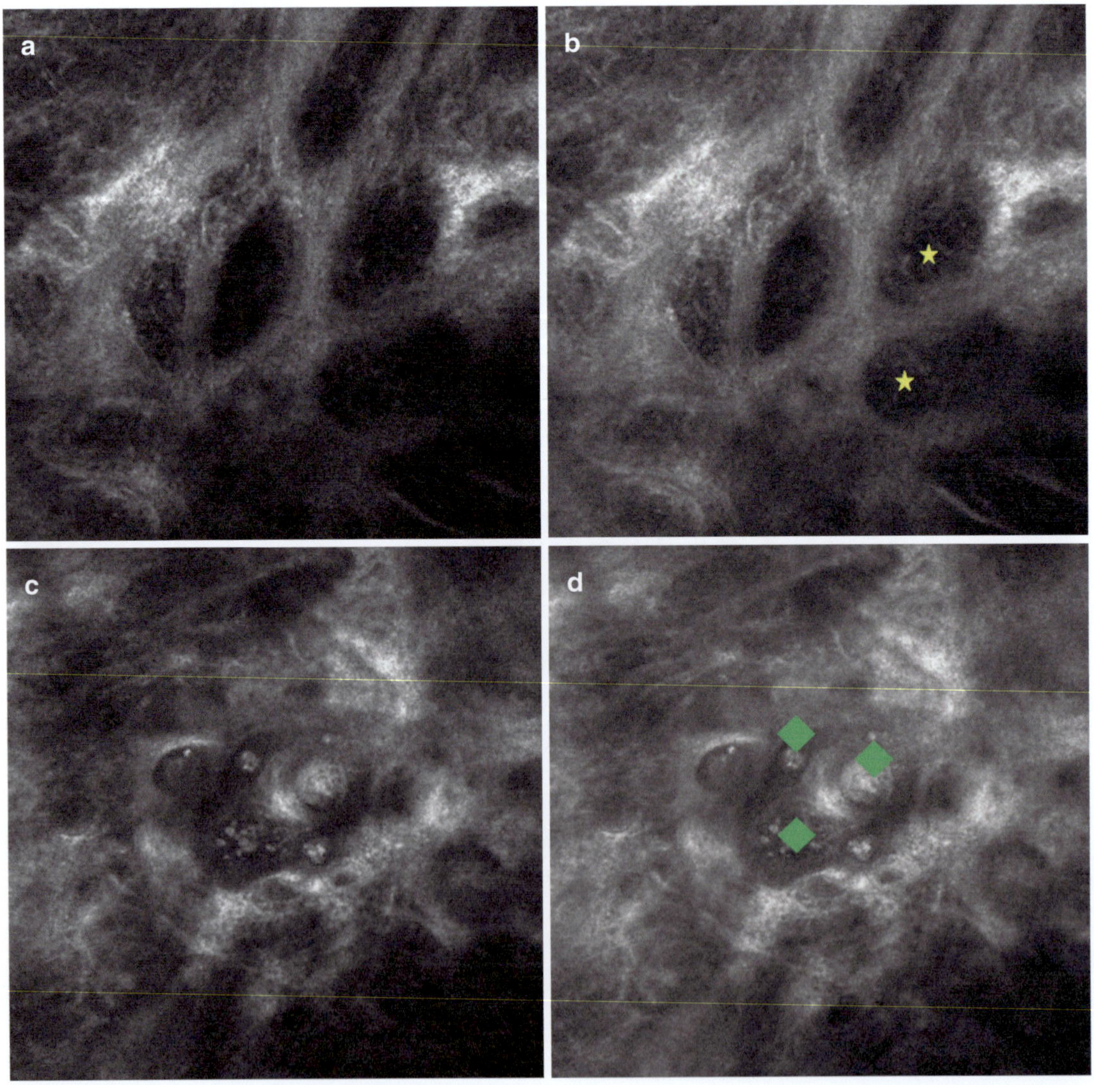

Fig. 10.8 IVCM features of syringoma (**a–d**)

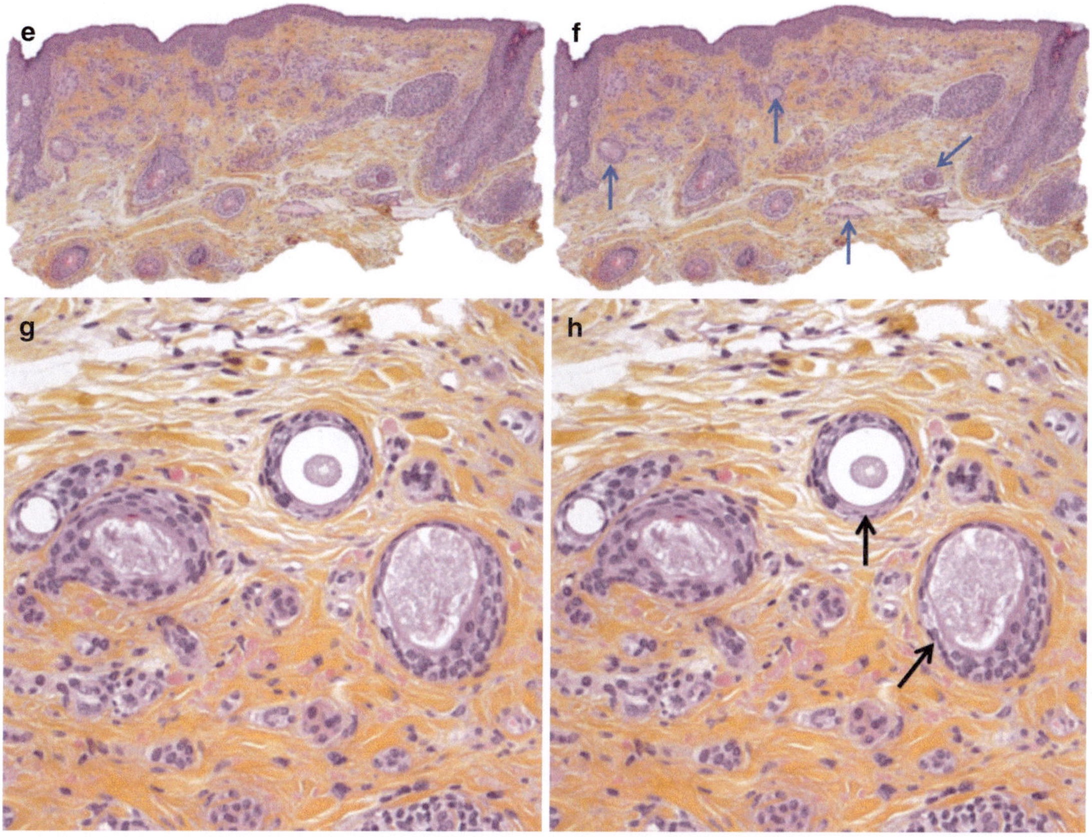

Fig. 10.9 Histological features of syringoma (**e–h**). (**e**, **f**) ×50 HES. (**g**, **h**) ×200 HES

On optical microscopy the histologic features are as follows (Fig. 10.9e–h):

- At low magnification (e, f), eccrine ductal structures are seen in the dermis (*blue arrows*).
- At high magnification (g, h), these tubular formations are bordered by a double layer of epithelial cells (*black arrows*).

10.2 Sebaceous Adenocarcinoma

Sebaceous adenocarcinoma is a rare malignant tumor developed mainly from the sebaceous glands of Meibomian.

The clinical aspect (Fig. 10.10) of sebaceous adenocarcinoma is that of an atypical chalazion increasing in size. Madarosis may be present.

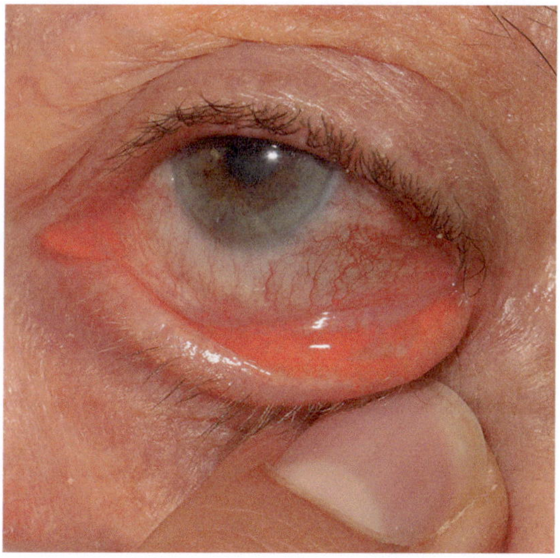

Fig. 10.10 Clinical aspect of sebaceous adenocarcinoma

The IVCM features are as follows (Fig. 10.11a–d):

- Normal tarsal conjunctival coating is seen (not shown here).
- Here, the free edge of the eyelid margin is normal with hyperreflective keratin deposits on its surface (*red diamonds*).
- In underlying dermis, lobules of poorly reflecting cells (*blue dotted lines*) are contoured by hyperreflective stroma (*yellow star*).

Under IVCM it is possible to assess that this tumor has a sebaceous origin, but it is not possible to observe cell details that prove its malignancy.

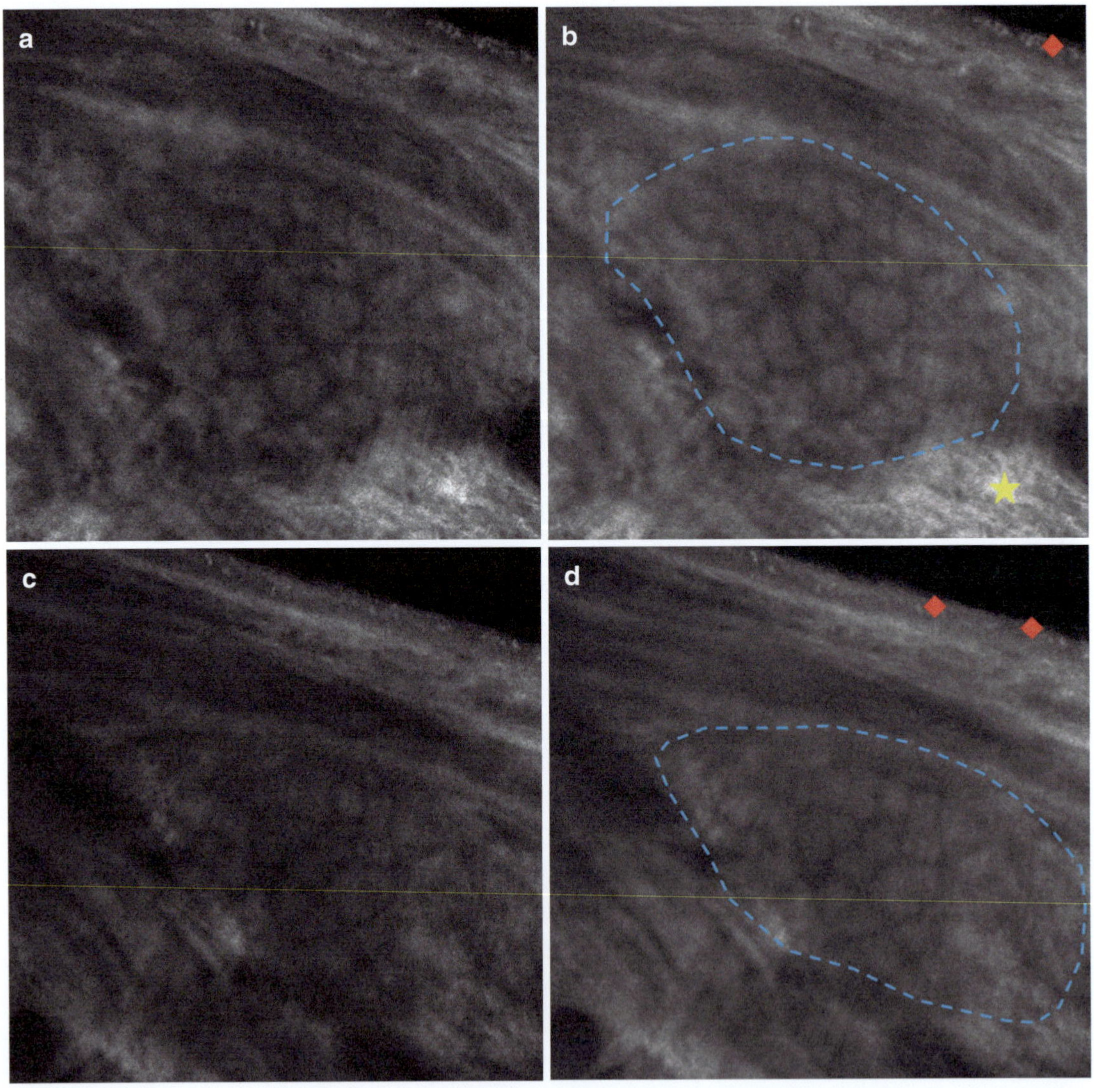

Fig. 10.11 IVCM features of sebaceous adenocarcinoma (**a–d**)

On optical microscopy the histologic features are as follows (Fig. 10.12e–h):

- At low magnification (e, f), the tumor proliferation (*black diamonds*) is basophilic with polycyclic contours, and infiltrates the dermis in the deeper layers (the epidermis is respected). The cells can extend deeply and often involve the subcutaneous tissue and even the underlying muscle. Fatty acid crystals (*orange stars*) are visible.
- At high magnification (g, h), poorly differentiated tumor cells are visible. The cells show variable sebaceous differentiation: there are normal-looking sebaceous cells (*red dotted line*) and pleomorphic cells with basophilic cytoplasm, and atypical and dysmorphic nuclei with abnormal mitoses (*black arrows*). Nuclei are usually large, with large nucleoli. The stroma is not well formed (*green crosses*).

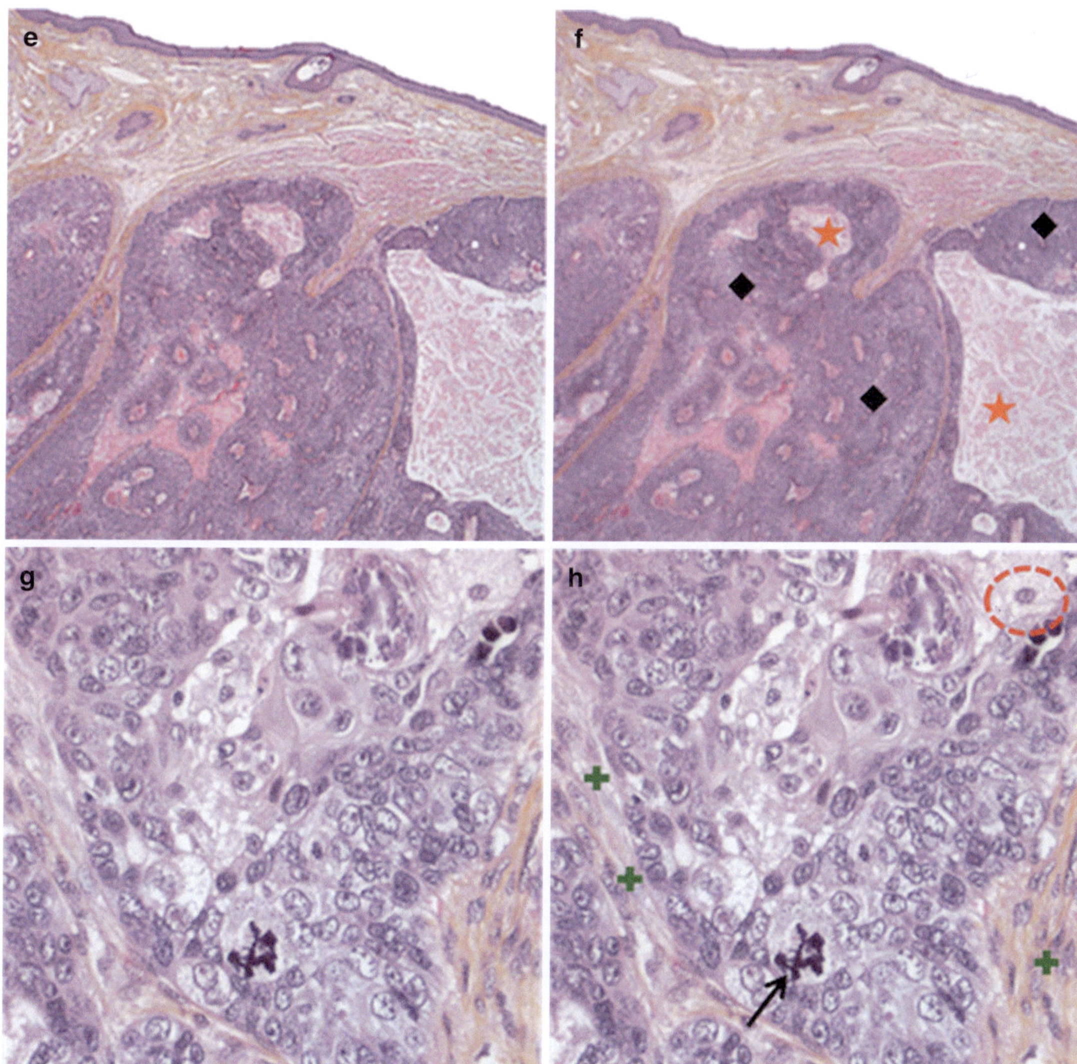

Fig. 10.12 Histological features of sebaceous adenocarcinoma (**e–h**). (**e, f**) ×25 HES. (**g, h**) ×400 HES

Vascular Tumors 11

Mathilde Kaspi, Thibaud Garcin, Elisa Cinotti,
Damien Grivet, Cyril Habougit,
and Jean-Luc Perrot

Content

Abbreviations

HES	Hematoxylin-eosin-saffron stain
IVCM	In vivo reflectance confocal microscopy

M. Kaspi (✉) · T. Garcin · D. Grivet
Department of Ophthalmology, University Hospital of Saint-Etienne, Saint-Etienne, France
e-mail: mathilde.kaspi@gmail.com; garcinthibaud@gmail.com; damien.grivet@chu-st-etienne.fr

E. Cinotti
Department of Dermatology, University of Siena, S. Maria alle Scotte Hospital, Siena, Italy
e-mail: elisa.cinotti@unisi.it

C. Habougit
Department of Pathology, University Hospital of Saint-Etienne, Saint-Etienne, France
e-mail: cyril.habougit@chu-st-etienne.fr

J.-L. Perrot
Department of Dermatology, University Hospital of Saint-Etienne, Saint-Etienne, France
e-mail: j.luc.perrot@chu-st-etienne.fr

11.1 Cavernous Hemangioma

The clinical aspect (Fig. 11.1) of this vascular lesion is a bluish-purple papule.

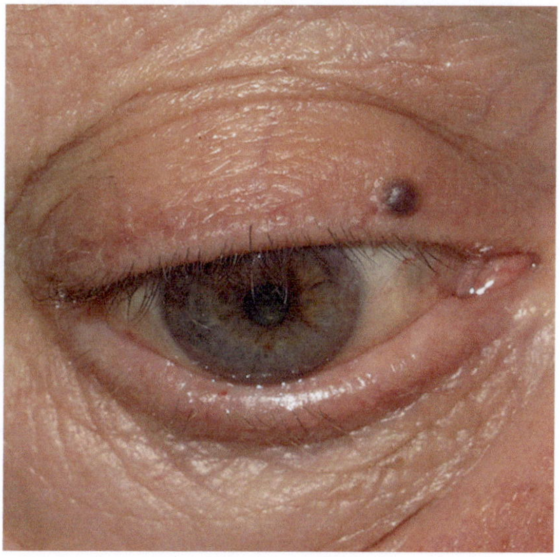

Fig. 11.1 Clinical aspect of cavernous hemangioma

© Springer Nature Switzerland AG 2020
M. Kaspi et al. (eds.), *Eyelid and Conjunctival Tumors*,
https://doi.org/10.1007/978-3-030-36606-3_11

The IVCM features are as follows (Fig. 11.2a–d):

– Normal epidermis and dermo-epidermal junction (not shown here)
– Large hyporeflective cavity (*orange arrows*) containing small hyperreflective cells (*yellow circle*) in the dermis.

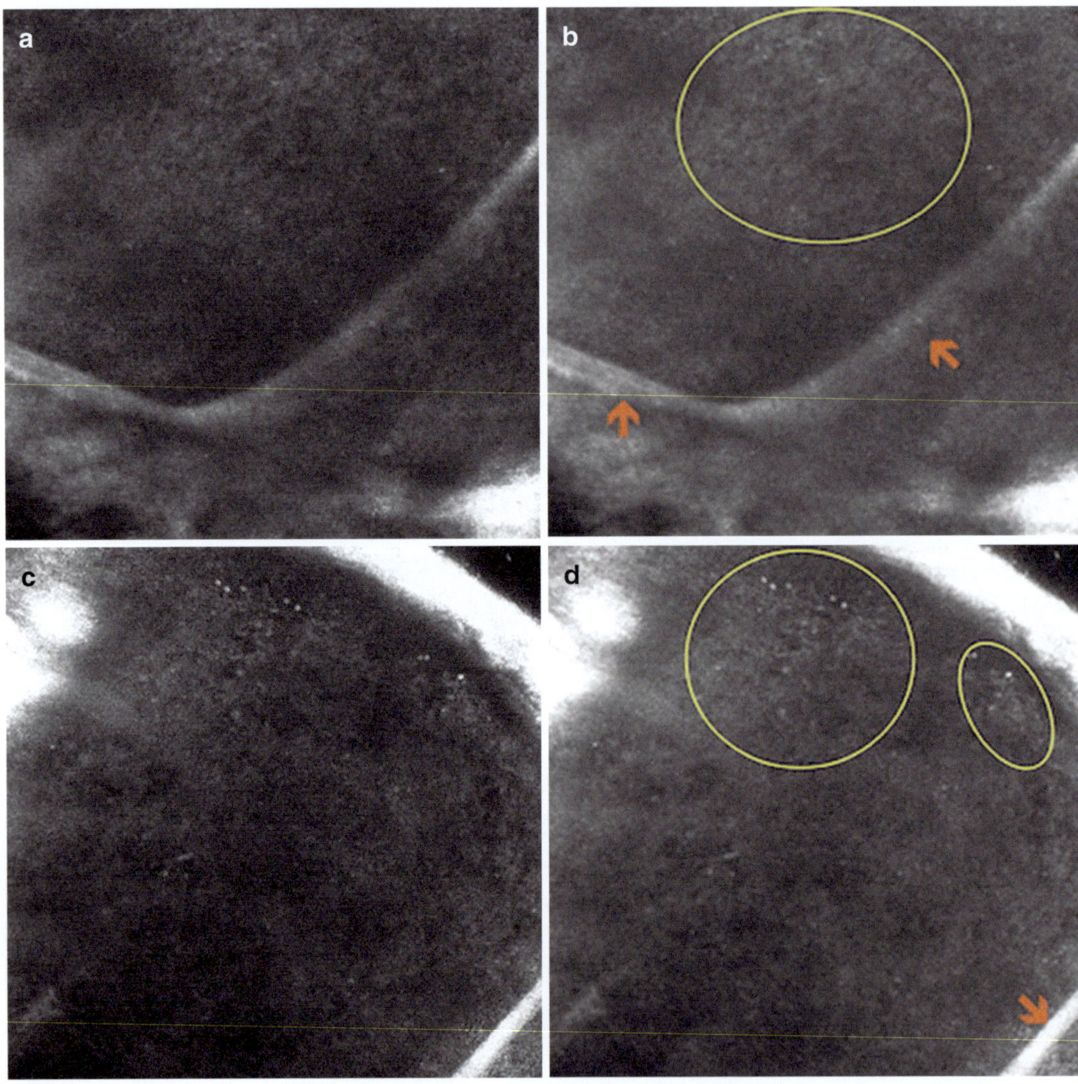

Fig. 11.2 IVCM features of cavernous hemangioma (**a–d**)

On optical microscopy the histologic features are as follows (Fig. 11.3e–h):

- Partially dilated thrombosed vessel (*grey crosses*) with cavernous arrangement
- The endothelial lining that is unevenly visible (*black arrows*)
- Old endoluminal and parietal thrombosis (*grey crosses*), accompanied by a significant inflammatory and siderophagic reaction (*yellow stars*)

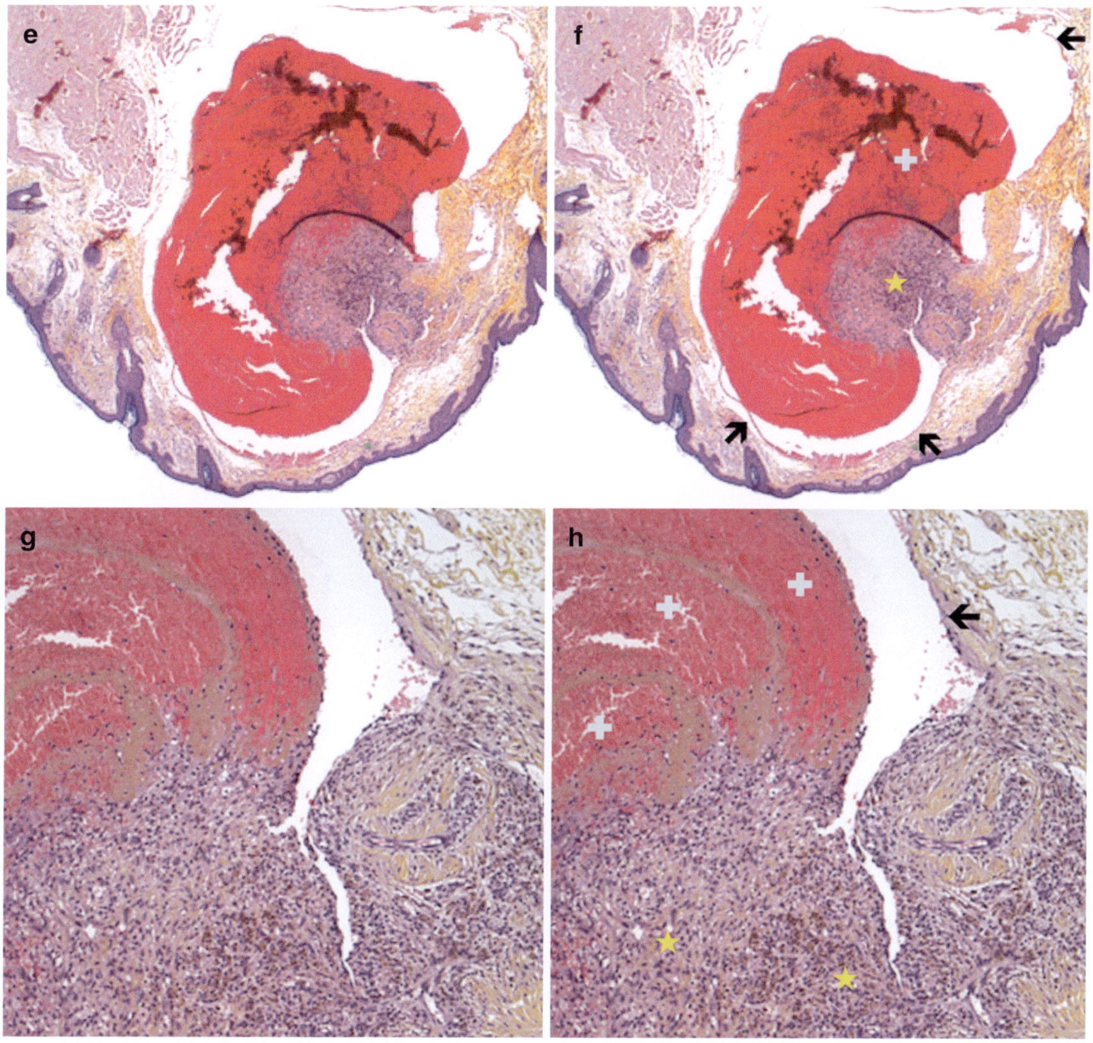

Fig. 11.3 Histological features of cavernous hemangioma (**e**–**h**). (**e**–**f**) ×25 HES. (**g**–**h**) ×100 HES

Miscellaneous Tumors

12

Mathilde Kaspi, Thibaud Garcin, Elisa Cinotti, Damien Grivet, Cyril Habougit, and Jean-Luc Perrot

Contents

Abbreviations

HES	Hematoxylin-eosin-saffron stain
IVCM	In vivo reflectance confocal microscopy

M. Kaspi (✉) · T. Garcin · D. Grivet
Department of Ophthalmology, University Hospital of Saint-Etienne, Saint-Etienne, France
e-mail: mathilde.kaspi@gmail.com; garcinthibaud@gmail.com; damien.grivet@chu-st-etienne.fr

E. Cinotti
Department of Dermatology, University of Siena, S. Maria alle Scotte Hospital, Siena, Italy
e-mail: elisa.cinotti@unisi.it

C. Habougit
Department of Pathology, University Hospital of Saint-Etienne, Saint-Etienne, France
e-mail: cyril.habougit@chu-st-etienne.fr

J.-L. Perrot
Department of Dermatology, University Hospital of Saint-Etienne, Saint-Etienne, France
e-mail: j.luc.perrot@chu-st-etienne.fr

© Springer Nature Switzerland AG 2020
M. Kaspi et al. (eds.), *Eyelid and Conjunctival Tumors*,
https://doi.org/10.1007/978-3-030-36606-3_12

12.1 Non-lymphoid Cutaneous Infiltrates (Xanthelasma)

Xanthelasma is a benign non-Langerhans cell histiocytic dermal tumor. Hyperlipidemia may be associated.

Clinically (Fig. 12.1), xanthelasma is a pale yellow, slightly raised or flat lesion placed on the eyelids.

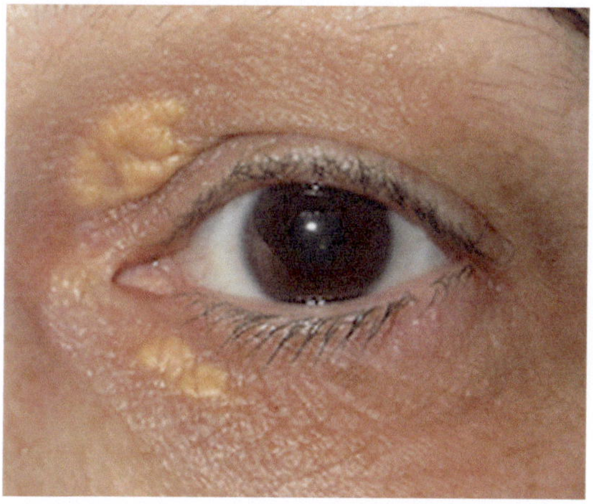

Fig. 12.1 Clinical aspect of xanthelasma

The IVCM features are as follows (Fig. 12.2a–d):

- Normal epidermis with regular honeycomb epidermis pattern (*red stars*)
- Normal dermo-epidermal junction (*yellow diamonds*)
- The lesion too deep to be visualized

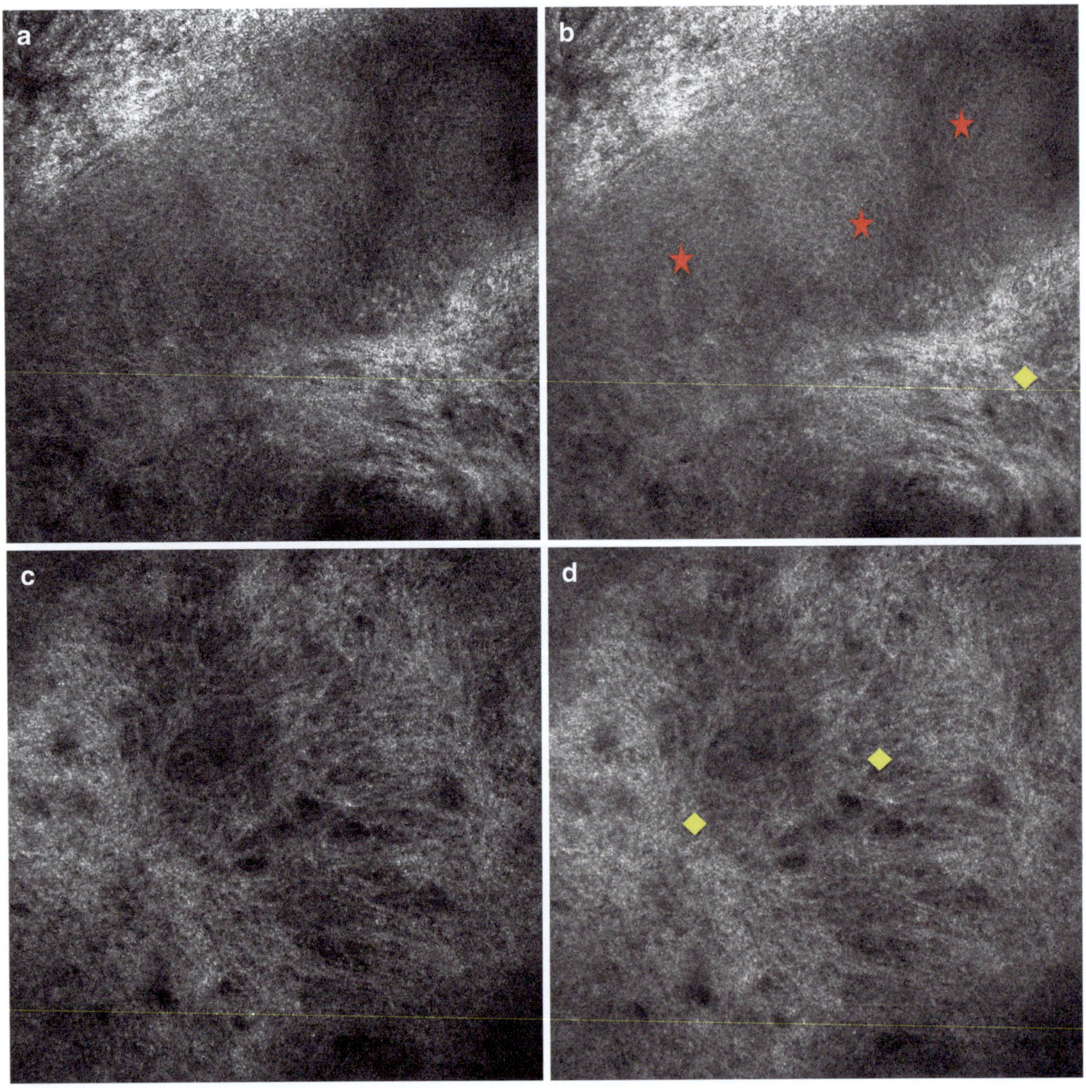

Fig. 12.2 IVCM features of xanthelasma (**a**–**d**)

On optical microscopy the histologic features are as follows (Fig. 12.3e–h):

- At low magnification (e, f), dermal foamy histiocytic elements (*black stars*) can be seen. The epidermis is normal.
- At high magnification (g, h), histiocytes (*black arrows*) have a large, vacuolized, light-colored cytoplasm associated with lipid accumulation.

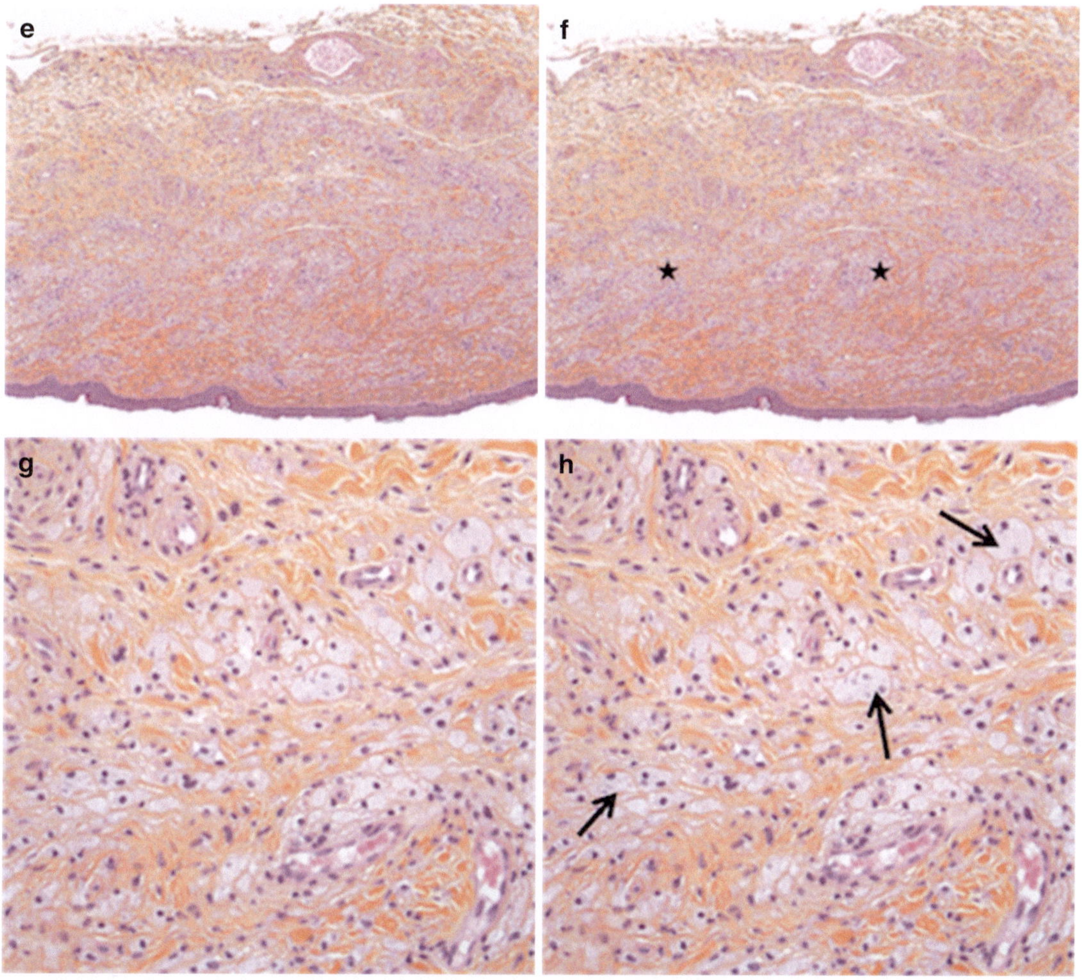

Fig. 12.3 Histological features of xanthelasma (**e**–**h**). (**e**–**f**) ×50 HES. (**g**–**h**) ×200 HES

12.2 Chalazion

Chalazion is secondary to an obstruction of the Meibomian ducts and corresponds to the resorptive granulomatous inflammation of the partially destroyed Meibomian sebaceous glands.

The clinical aspect of a chalazion is an inflammatory and painful swelling protruding from the cutaneous (Fig. 12.4) or conjunctival tarsal side. No madarosis is present.

The IVCM features are as follows (Fig. 12.5a–d):

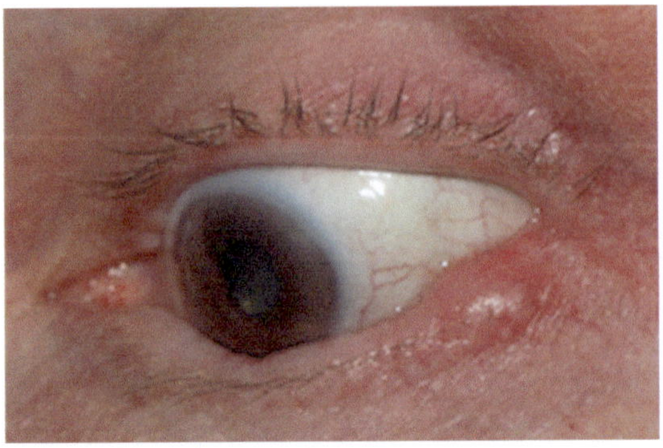

Fig. 12.4 Clinical aspect of chalazion

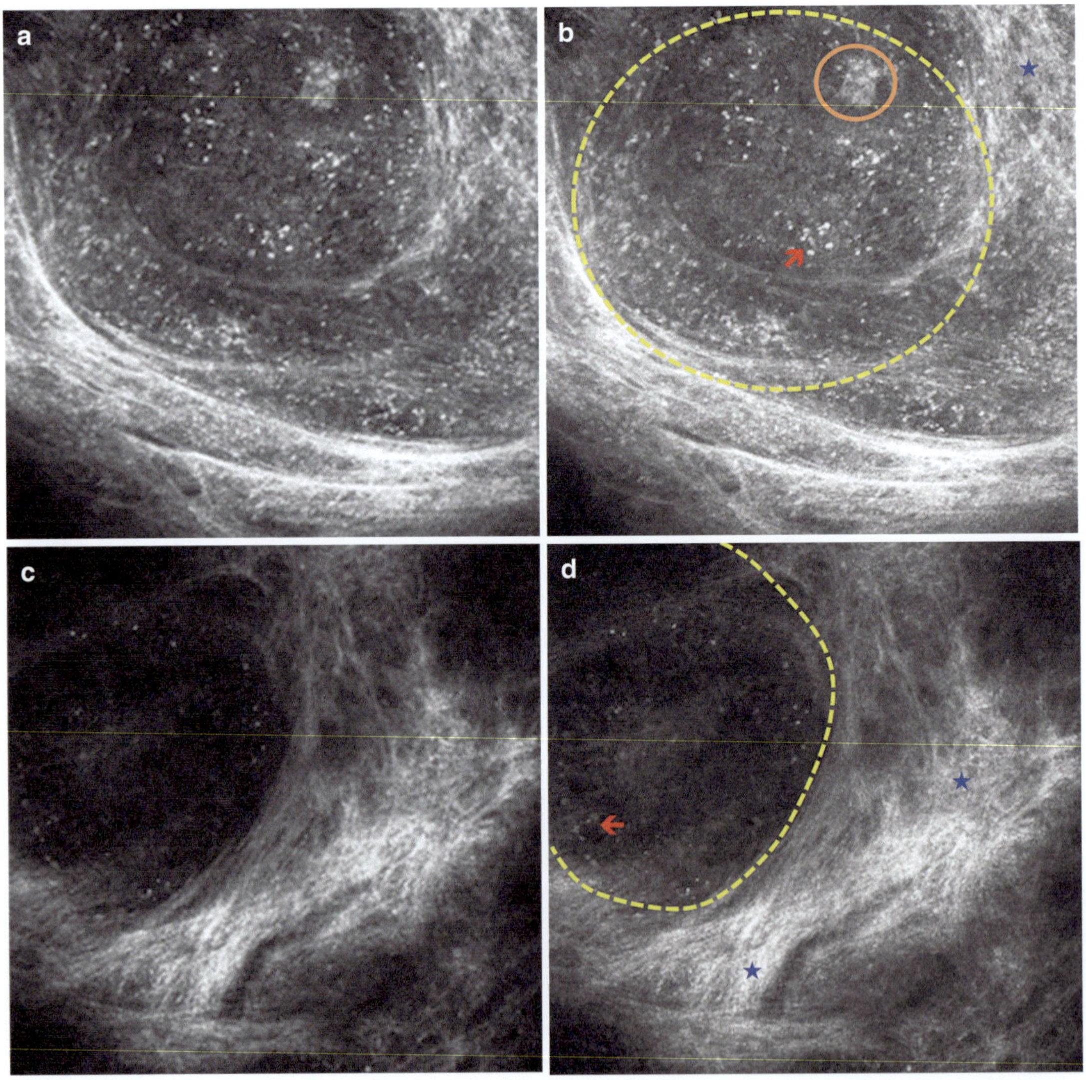

Fig. 12.5 IVCM features of chalazion (**a**–**d**)

- Normal epidermis with regular honeycomb epidermis pattern can be seen (not shown here).
- In superficial dermis, the Meibomian glands are dilated (*yellow dotted line*) and sometimes contain reflecting material (*orange circle*) representing the accumulation of meibum and inflammatory cells (*red arrows*). These glands are surrounded by fibrous structures (*blue stars*).

On optical microscopy the histologic features are as follows (Fig. 12.6e–h):

- At low magnification (e–f), the granulomatous inflammation in the tarsus (*blue line*) is centered around a dystrophic and dilated Meibomian gland (*black arrows*). An unscathed Meibomian gland (*black stars*) and the orbicular muscle (*green diamonds*) are visible.
- At high magnification (g–h), the optically empty spaces correspond to the lipids dissolved by solvents during the inclusion steps. The inflammatory reaction is heavy without gigantocellular cells in this example.

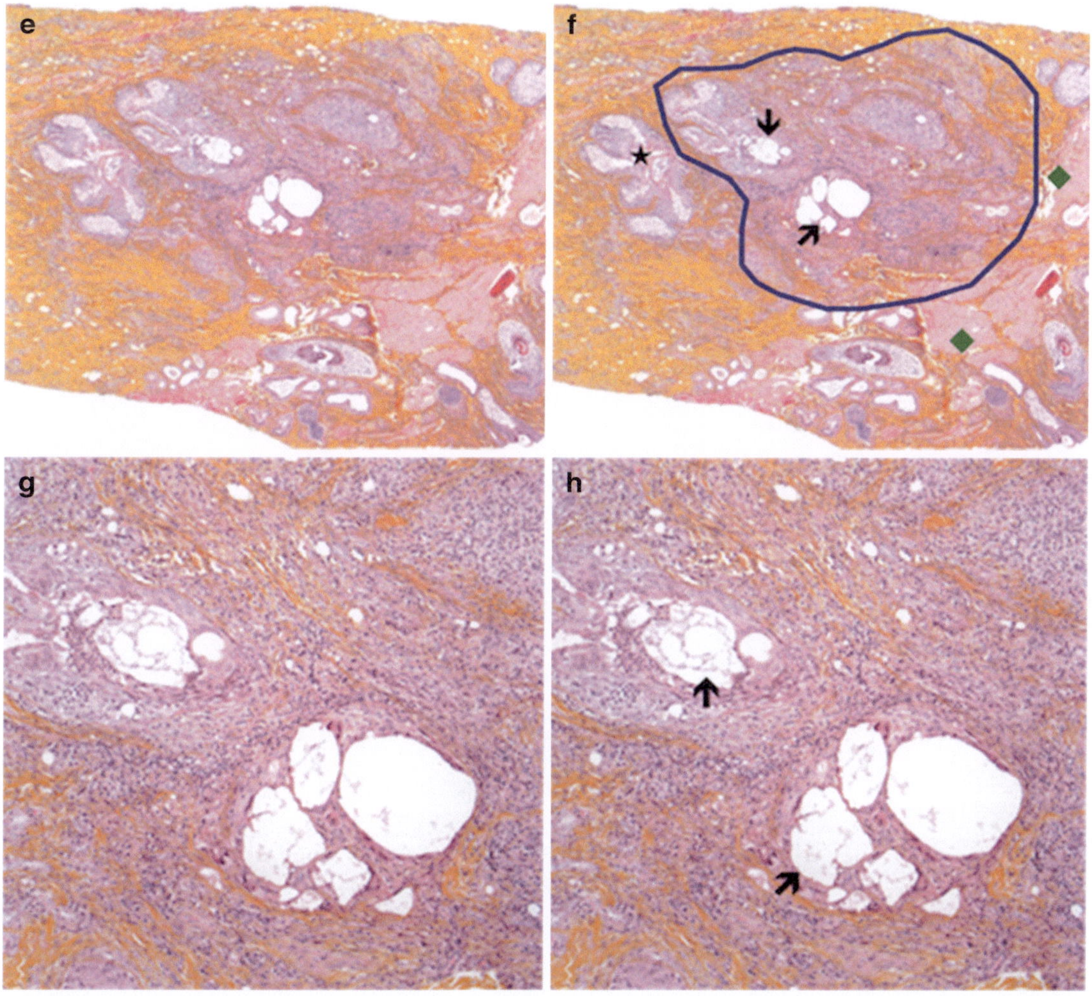

Fig. 12.6 Histological features of chalazion (**e**–**h**). (**e**–**f**) ×25 HES. (**g**–**h**) ×100 HES

12.3 Stye

Stye is an inflammatory and painful papulopustule of the eyelid margin associated with staphylococcal infection. An eyelash may be present in the pustule.

Clinically (Fig. 12.7), a stye is an erythematous papule or a pustule with an erythematous background located on the eyelid margin.

In IVCM (Fig. 12.8a–d), the dilated hair follicle (*red star*) is surrounded by large hyperreflective inflammatory cells corresponding to histiocytes (*blue line*).

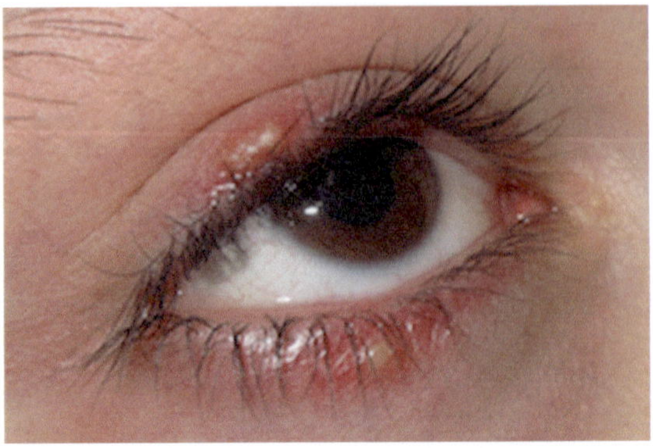

Fig. 12.7 Clinical aspect of stye

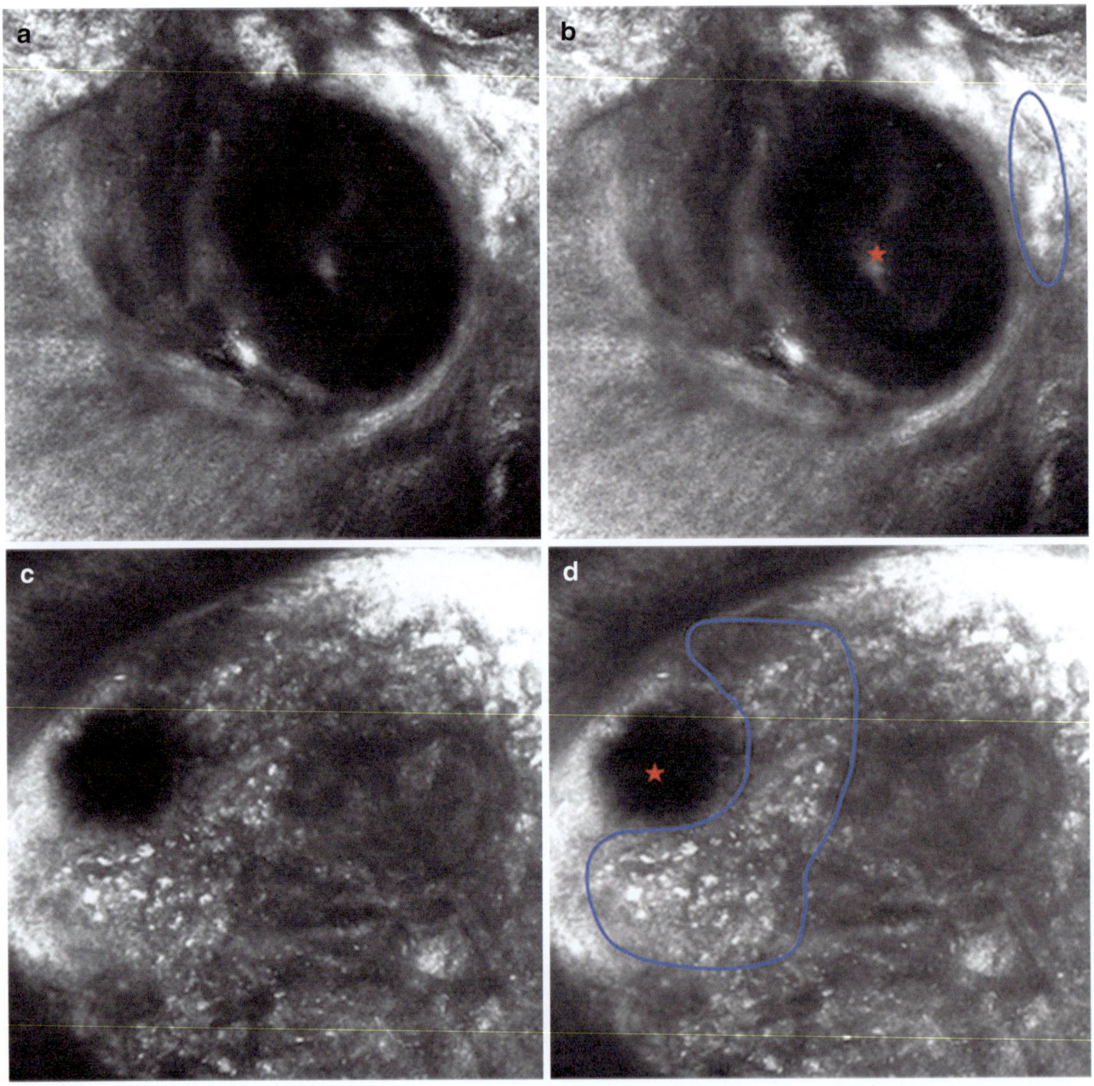

Fig. 12.8 IVCM features of stye (**a**–**d**)

On optical microscopy (Fig. 12.9e–h), in this case acute perifollicular dermal inflammation (*black stars*) involves two adjacent pilosebaceous follicles (*blue circles*). The pilosebaceous follicles show cystic dilation of their infundibulum. The Zeis sebaceous glands (*green arrows*) adjacent to the hair follicles and the Moll sweat glands (*orange diamond*) located between the follicles are visible.

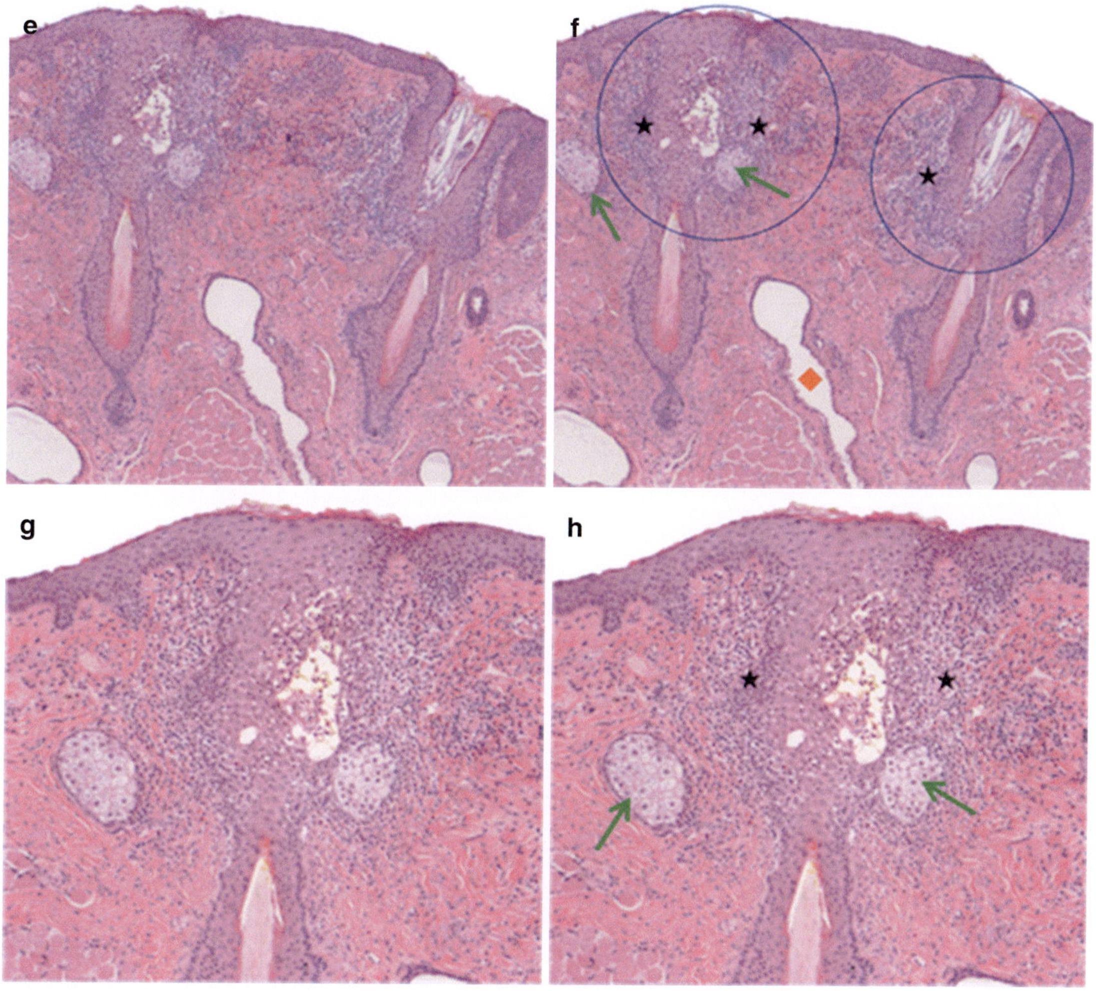

Fig. 12.9 Histological features of stye (**e**–**h**). (**e**–**f**) ×50 HES. (**g**–**h**) ×100 HES

Part V

Conjunctival Tumors

Epithelial Conjunctival Tumors

13

Thibaud Garcin, Mathilde Kaspi, Cyril Habougit, Damien Grivet, Jean-Luc Perrot, and Elisa Cinotti

Contents

Abbreviations

Ab	Antibodies
HES	Hematoxylin-eosin-saffron stain
IVCM	In vivo reflectance confocal microscopy

T. Garcin (✉) · M. Kaspi · D. Grivet
Department of Ophthalmology, University Hospital of Saint-Etienne, Saint-Etienne, France
e-mail: garcinthibaud@gmail.com; mathilde.kaspi@gmail.com; damien.grivet@chu-st-etienne.fr

C. Habougit
Department of Pathology, University Hospital of Saint-Etienne, Saint-Etienne, France
e-mail: cyril.habougit@chu-st-etienne.fr

J.-L. Perrot
Department of Dermatology, University Hospital of Saint-Etienne, Saint-Etienne, France
e-mail: j.luc.perrot@chu-st-etienne.fr

E. Cinotti
Department of Dermatology, University of Siena, S. Maria alle Scotte Hospital, Siena, Italy
e-mail: elisa.cinotti@unisi.it

13.1 Epithelial Dysplasia

Epithelial dysplasia can be flat or raised. Here (Fig. 13.1) the patient presents a white, budding raised lesion with a feeder vessel (*black arrow*).

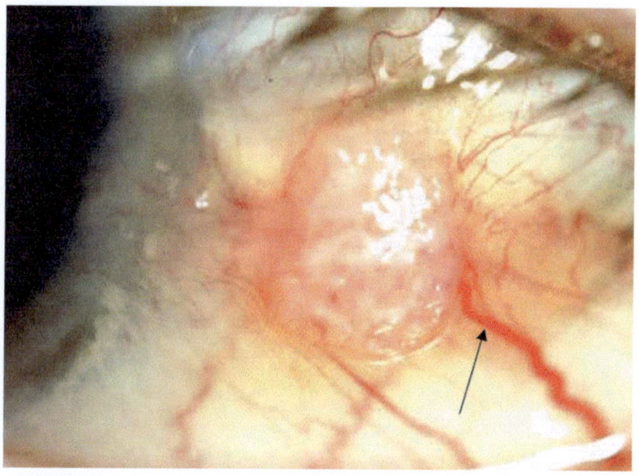

Fig. 13.1 Clinical aspect of epithelial dysplasia: slit-lamp photography

© Springer Nature Switzerland AG 2020
M. Kaspi et al. (eds.), *Eyelid and Conjunctival Tumors*,
https://doi.org/10.1007/978-3-030-36606-3_13

The IVCM features are as follows (Fig. 13.2a–d):

- Disorganization of the conjunctival epithelium with cells of variable size and reflectance (*blue stars*) can be seen.
- Cell roll (*red dotted line*) and images of pseudo-epithelial cavities are visible (*yellow arrows*).
- The lower and median layers of the epithelium show cytological atypia; the superficial layers keep maturation without dyskeratosis.

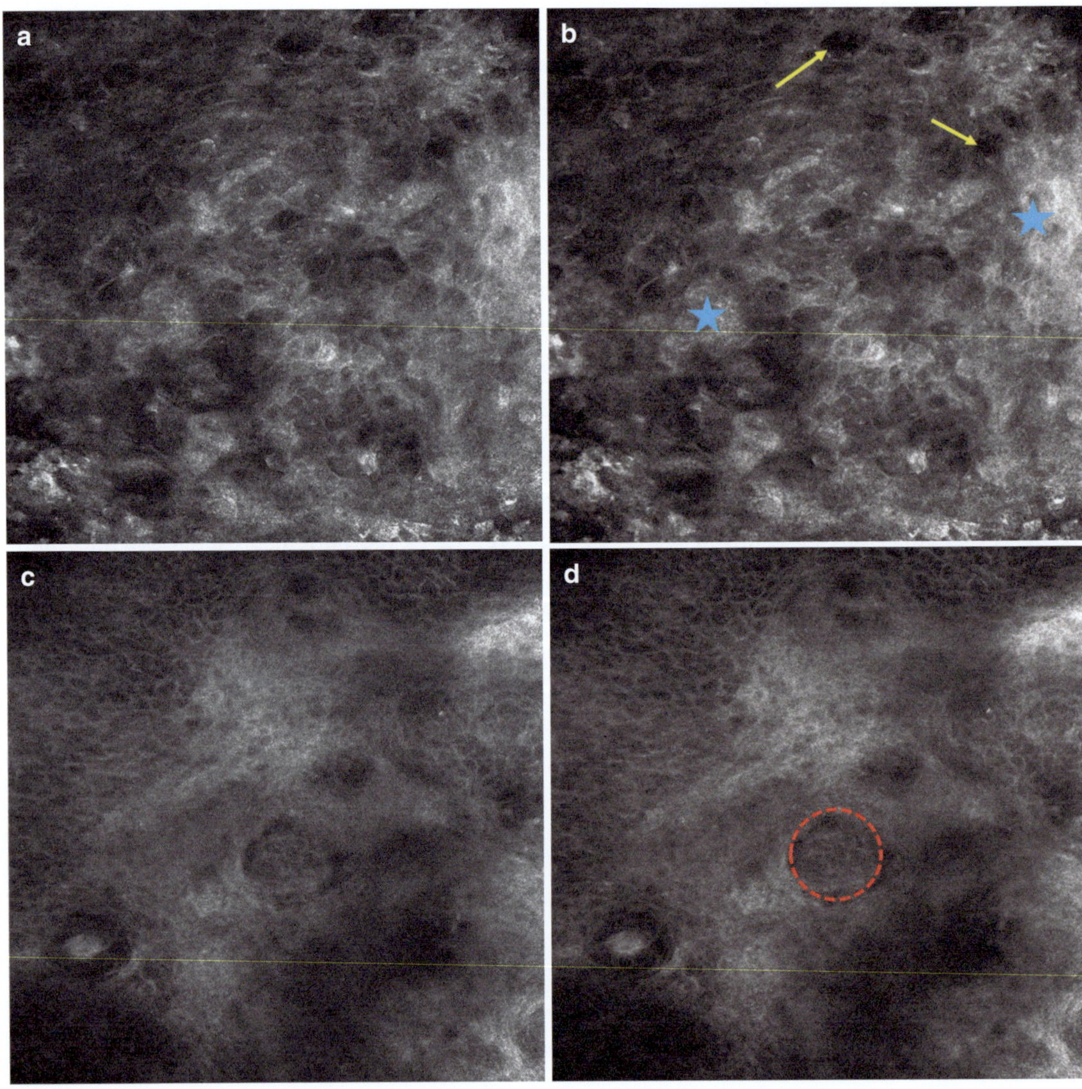

Fig. 13.2 IVCM features of epithelial dysplasia (**a**–**d**)

On optical microscopy the histologic features are as follows (Fig. 13.3e–h):

- At low magnification (e–f), in this case the proliferation of the squamous epithelium is exophytic. Epithelial hyperplasia is arranged in anastomotic cords containing islands of connective tissue (*black stars*) and keratin pearl pseudocysts (*blue arrows*).
- At high magnification (g–h), the basement membrane does not show any alteration. The lower and median layers of the epithelium include cytonuclear atypia (*yellow circle*). The superficial layers keep maturation without dyskeratosis.

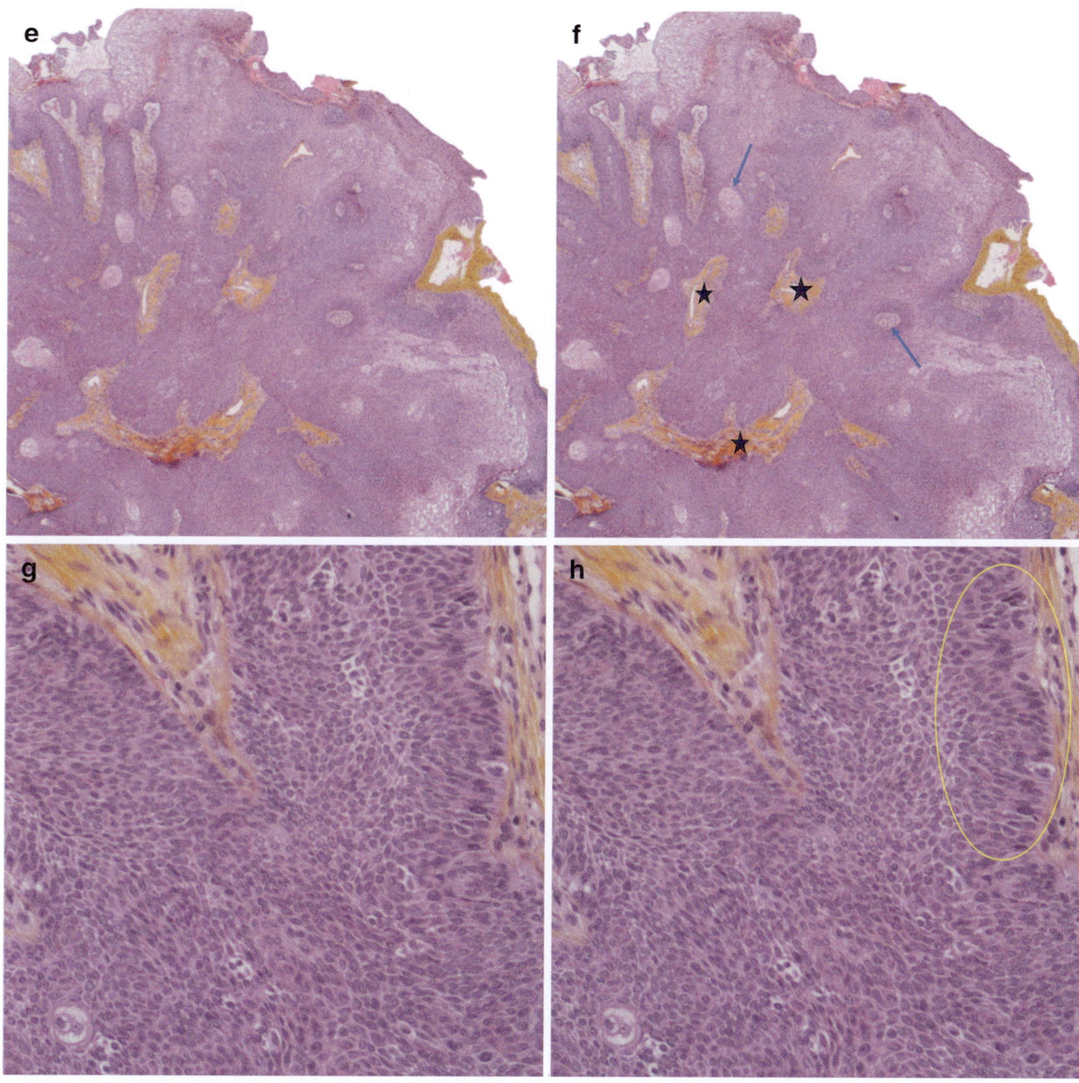

Fig. 13.3 Histological features of epithelial dysplasia (**e**–**h**). (**e, f**) ×25HES. (**g, h**) ×200 HES

13.2 Squamous Cell Carcinoma

Ultraviolet exposure is a major risk factor for squamous cell carcinoma.

Squamous cell carcinoma can occur in different clinical forms: leukoplakia, gelatinous, papillomatous, pedunculated, nodular, and diffuse. The diffuse form very often mimics a chronic conjunctivitis. Limbal involvement and orbital invasion are possible. Squamous cell carcinoma in situ is limited to the entire epithelium, whereas invasive squamous cell carcinoma crosses the basal membrane of the epithelium and invades the chorion.

13.2.1 In Situ Squamous Cell Carcinoma: Gelatinous Form

The clinical aspect (Fig. 13.4a–b) of a gelatinous squamous cell carcinoma is that of a whitish lesion with a wet sugar appearance. Here the lesion is surrounded by dilated superficial feeder vessels (*yellow circle*) and the limbus is invaded.

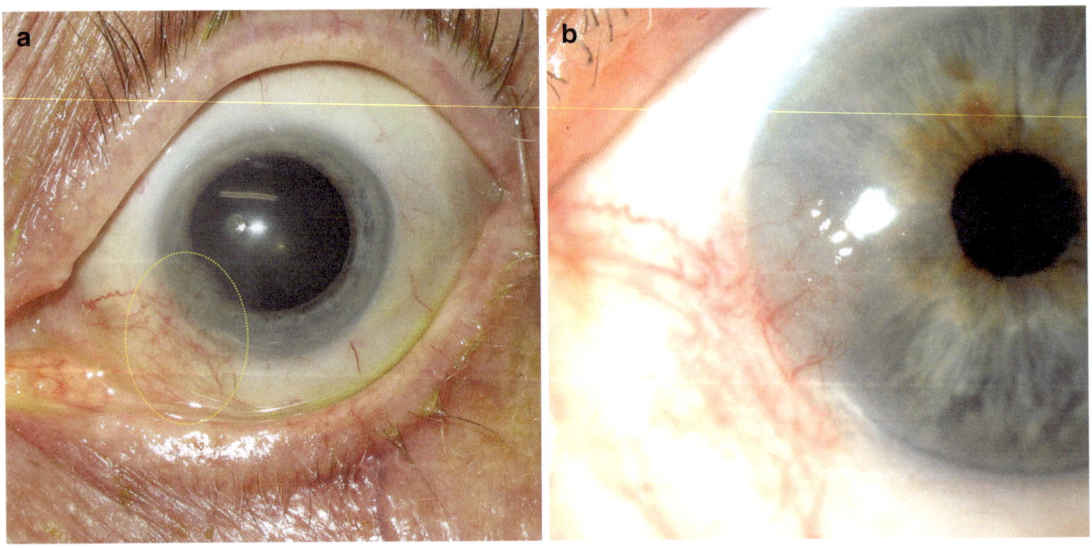

Fig. 13.4 Clinical aspect of in situ gelatinous form of squamous cell carcinoma: macroscopic photography (**a**) and slit-lamp photography (**b**)

The IVCM features are as follows (Fig. 13.5c–f):

- Corneal epithelium at the level of the limbus is disorganized (*yellow diamond*), instead of having the regular honeycomb pattern (*green diamond*) of the normal cornea.
- Conjunctival epithelium is thickened and disorganized (*blue stars*).
- Tumor lobules show roll-up pattern (*red dotted line*).

On optical microscopy the histologic features are as follows (Fig. 13.6g–l):

- At low magnification (g–k) the squamous proliferation (*black stars*) is intraepithelial.
- The tumor disorganizes the entire thickness of the epithelium, without crossing the basement epithelial membrane (*black line*). In immunohistochemistry, this proliferation is marked (in brown) by the anti-p53 antibody.
- At high magnification (k–l) atypical squamous cells have a large eosinophilic cytoplasm with some mitoses (*black arrows*). Abnormal drafts of squamous maturation are observed (*blue circles*). Parakeratosis is present on the surface (*green dotted lines*).

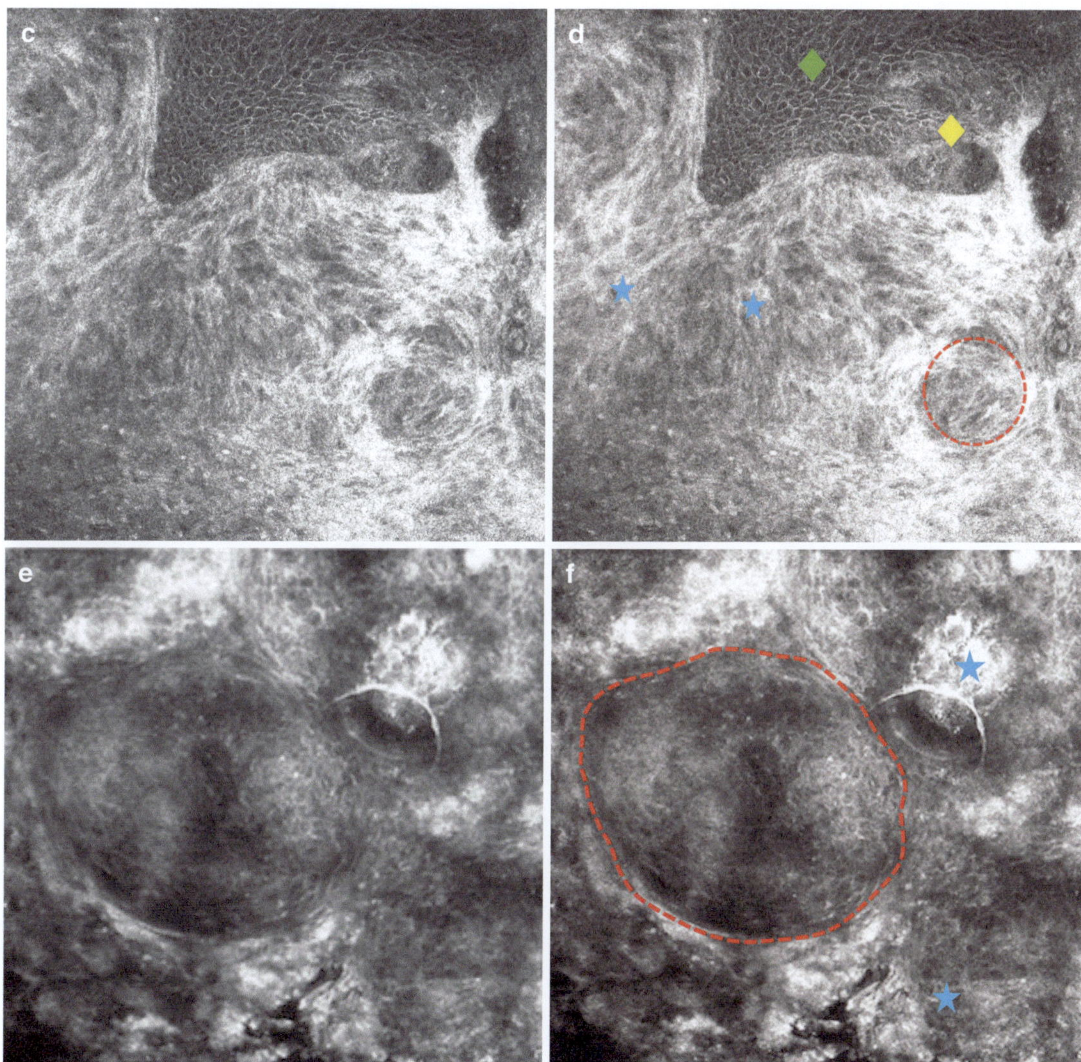

Fig. 13.5 IVCM features of in situ gelatinous form of squamous cell carcinoma (**c**–**f**)

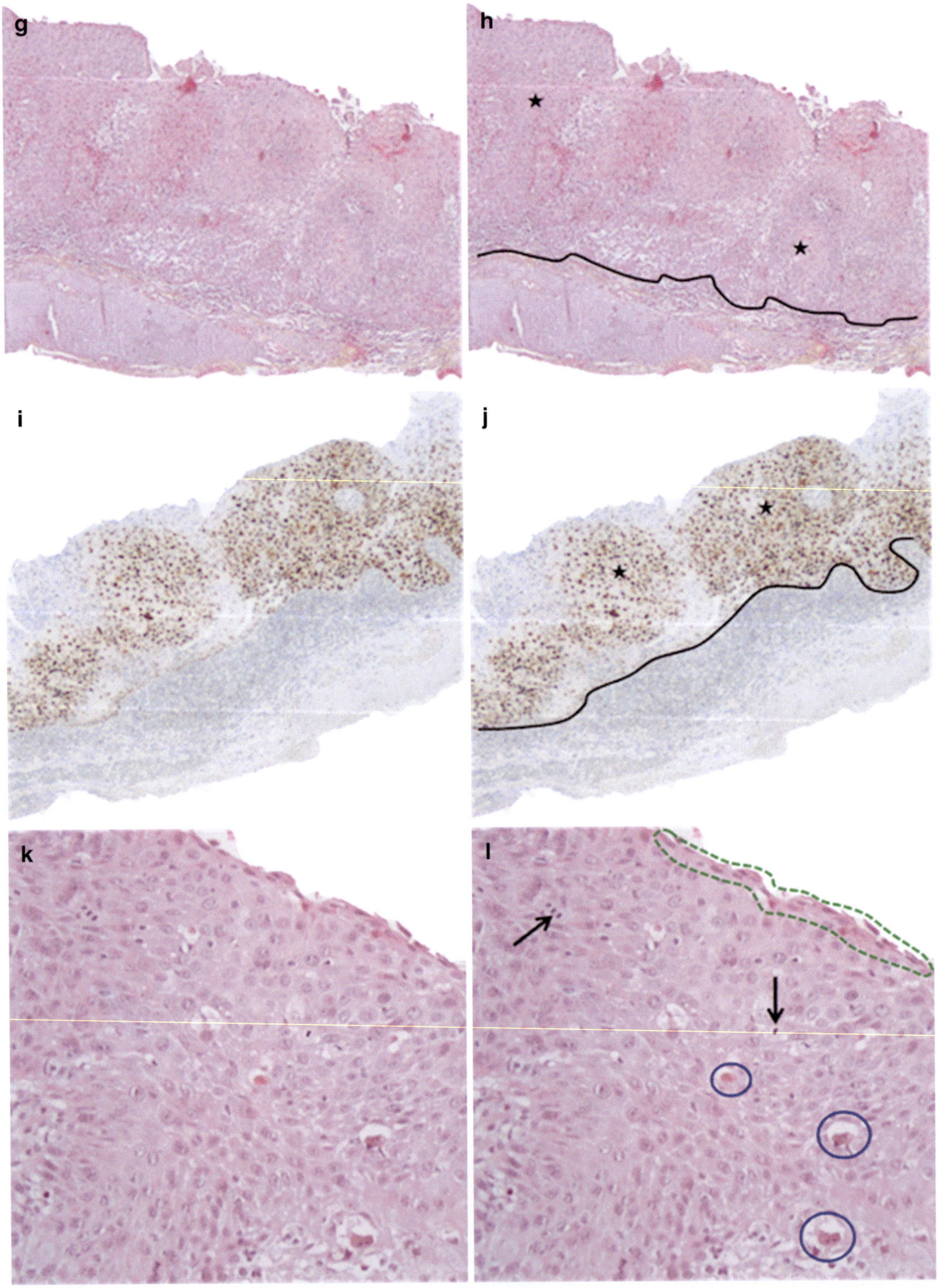

Fig. 13.6 Histological features of in situ gelatinous form of squamous cell carcinoma (**g–l**). (**g**, **h**) ×50 HES. (**i**, **j**) ×50 Anti-p53 Ab. (**k**, **l**) ×200 HES

13.2.2 In Situ Squamous Cell Carcinoma: Papillomatous Form

The papillomatous form (Fig. 13.7) is telangiectasic and more protruding. Dilated feeder vessels are visible (*black arrows*). The papillomatous form mimics conjunctival papilloma.

The IVCM features are as follows (Fig. 13.8a–d):

- Totally disorganized conjunctival epithelium is seen (*blue stars*).

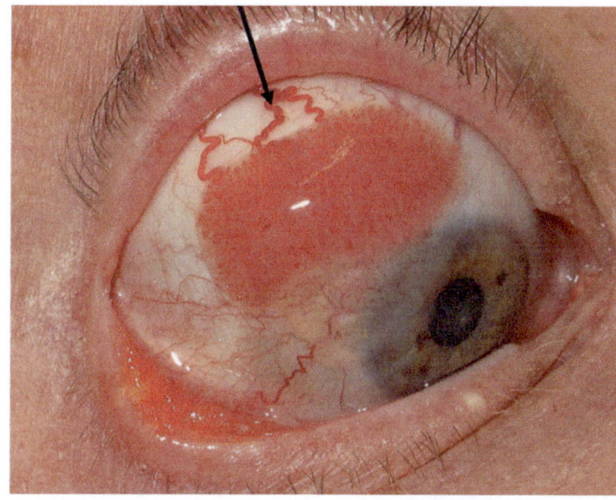

Fig. 13.7 Clinical aspect of in situ papillomatous form of squamous cell carcinoma

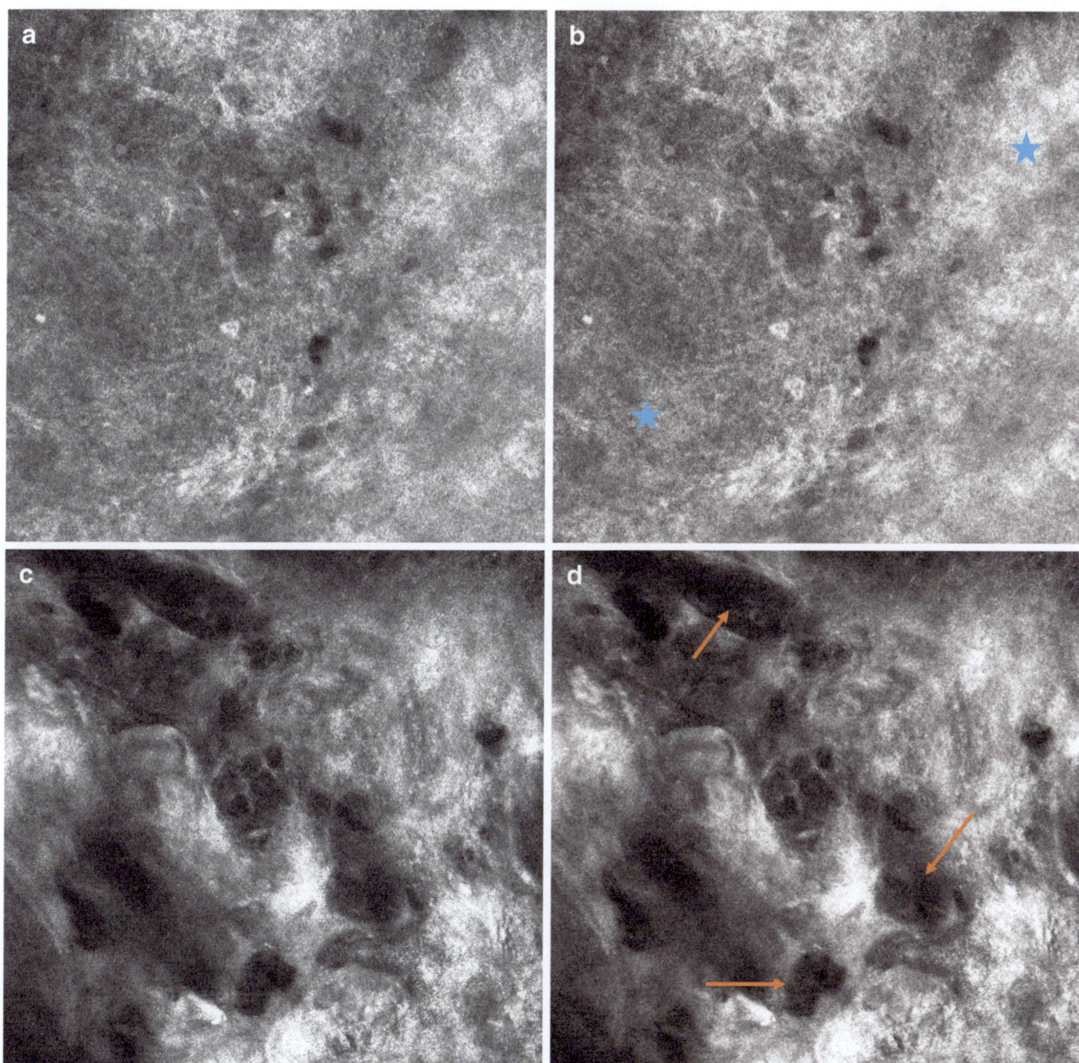

Fig. 13.8 IVCM features of in situ papillomatous form of squamous cell carcinoma (**a**–**d**)

– At greater depth, rounded hyporeflecting areas corresponding to the stroma (*orange arrows*) are visible; sometimes dilated vessels are often inside these areas.

On optical microscopy the histologic features are as follows (Fig. 13.9e–h):

– At low magnification (e–f), the proliferation of atypical squamous cells disrupts the architecture of the entire thickness of the epithelium, without crossing the basement membrane (*blue dotted lines*). Vessels are found within the proliferation (*green arrows*).
– At high magnification (g–h), proliferation is made up of joined polygonal cells with moderate atypia. Some mitoses are visible (*black arrows*).

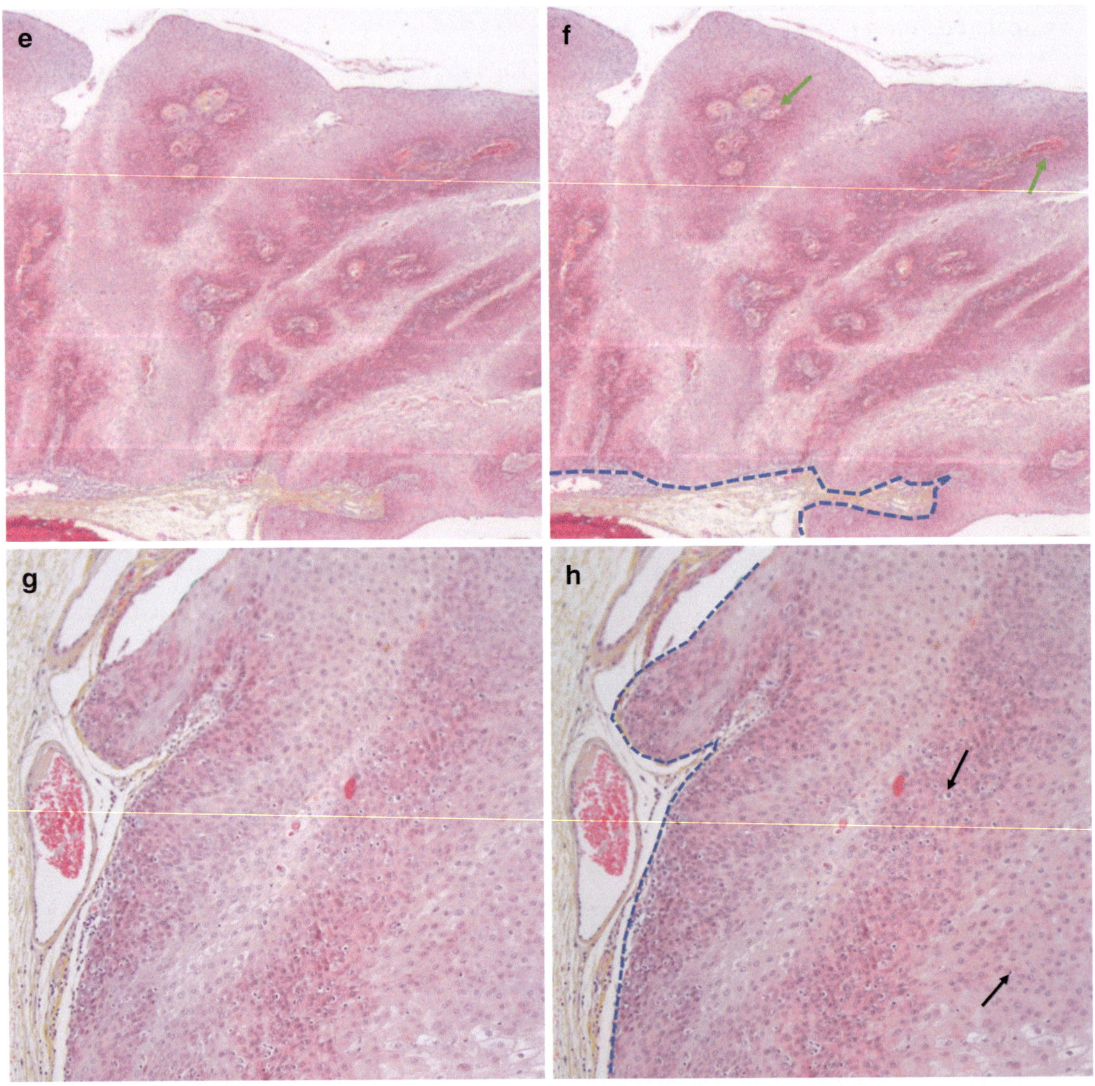

Fig. 13.9 Histological features of in situ papillomatous form of squamous cell carcinoma (**e**–**h**). (**e**, **f**) ×25 HES. (**g**, **h**) ×100 HES

13.2.3 Invasive Squamous Cell Carcinoma

This case of invasive squamous cell carcinoma is of gelatinous type with a wet sugar appearance (Fig. 13.10). It is surrounded by dilated superficial feeder vessels. The limbus is invaded.

The IVCM features are as follows (Fig. 13.11a–d):

– Corneal epithelium at the level of the limbus is disorganized (*yellow diamonds*), instead of having the regular honeycomb pattern (*green diamond*) of the normal cornea.

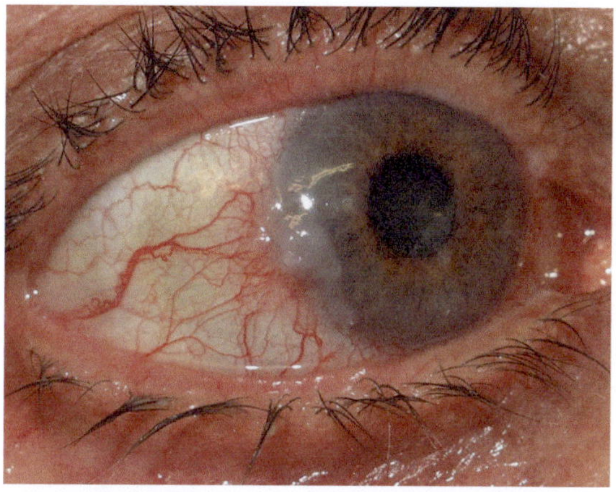

Fig. 13.10 Clinical aspect of invasive squamous cell carcinoma: slit-lamp photography

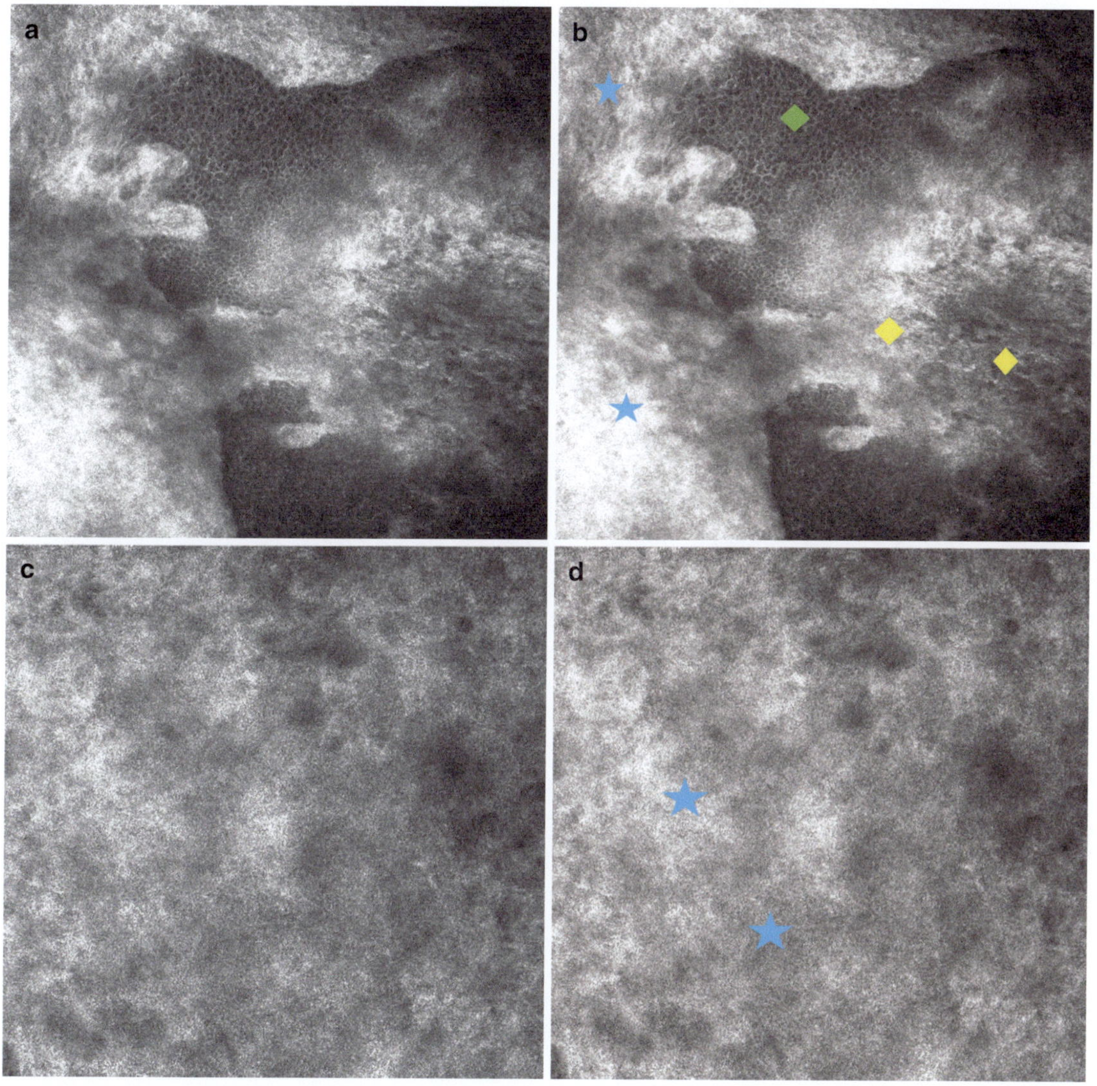

Fig. 13.11 IVCM features of invasive squamous cell carcinoma (**a–d**)

- Totally disorganized conjunctival epithelium is seen (*blue stars*).

On optical microscopy the histologic features are as follows (Fig. 13.12e–h):

- At low magnification (e, f), the proliferation of atypical squamous cells disrupts the architecture of the epithelium over its entire depth, with crossing of the basement membrane (*blue dotted lines*) and invasion of the chorionic layer (*blue arrow*).
- At high magnification (g, h), proliferation is made up of connected polygonal cells with high-grade cytonuclear atypia. Mitoses are visible (*black arrows*).

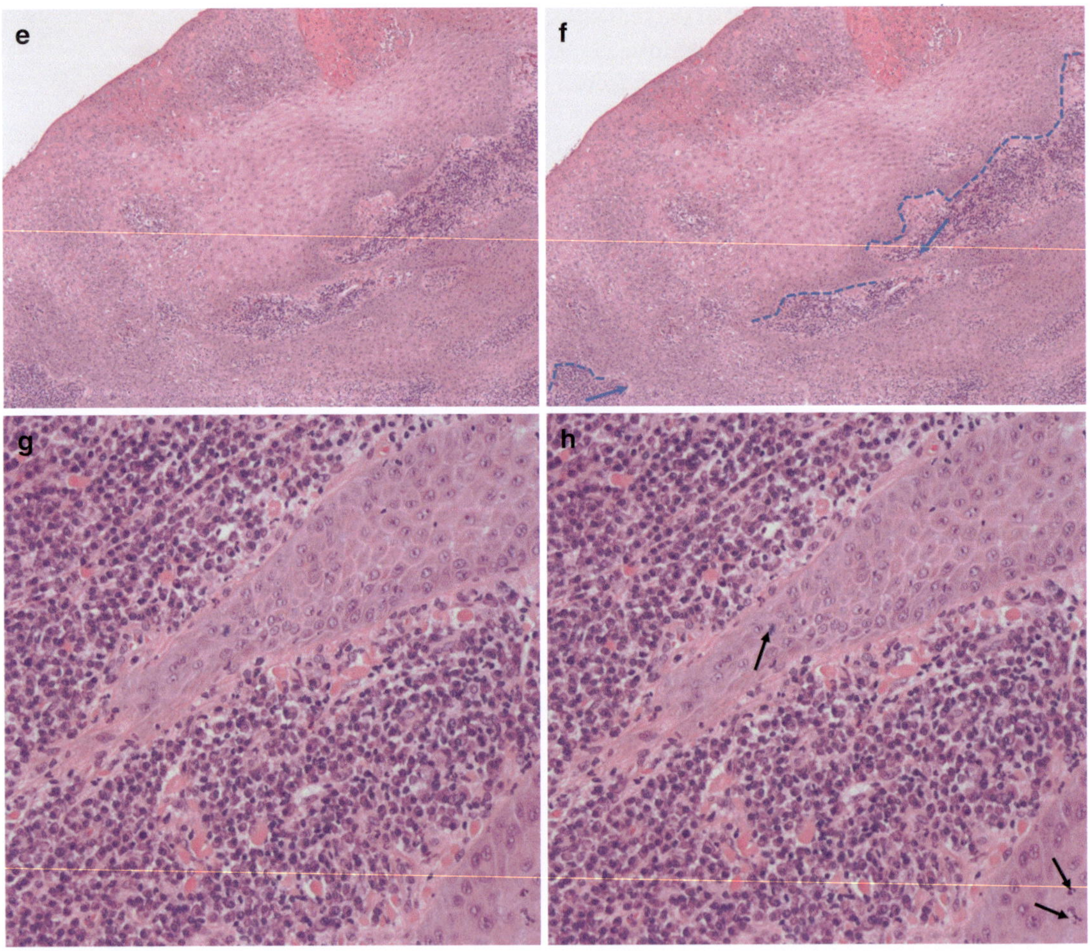

Fig. 13.12 Histological features of invasive squamous cell carcinoma (**e–h**). (**e**, **f**) ×50 HES. (**g**, **h**) ×200 HES

Melanocytic Conjunctival Tumors 14

Thibaud Garcin, Mathilde Kaspi, Cyril Habougit, Damien Grivet, Jean-Luc Perrot, and Elisa Cinotti

Contents

Abbreviations

Ab	Antibodies
HES	Hematoxylin-eosin-saffron stain
IVCM	In vivo reflectance confocal microscopy
PAM	Primary acquired melanosis

T. Garcin (✉) · M. Kaspi · D. Grivet
Department of Ophthalmology, University Hospital of Saint-Etienne, Saint-Etienne, France
e-mail: garcinthibaud@gmail.com; mathilde.kaspi@gmail.com; damien.grivet@chu-st-etienne.fr

C. Habougit
Department of Pathology, University Hospital of Saint-Etienne, Saint-Etienne, France
e-mail: cyril.habougit@chu-st-etienne.fr

J.-L. Perrot
Department of Dermatology, University Hospital of Saint-Etienne, Saint-Etienne, France
e-mail: j.luc.perrot@chu-st-etienne.fr

E. Cinotti
Department of Dermatology, University of Siena, S. Maria alle Scotte Hospital, Siena, Italy
e-mail: elisa.cinotti@unisi.it

© Springer Nature Switzerland AG 2020
M. Kaspi et al. (eds.), *Eyelid and Conjunctival Tumors*,
https://doi.org/10.1007/978-3-030-36606-3_14

14.1 Nevi

Depending on the location of the melanocyte proliferation, nevus is classified as

- Junctional (proliferation limited to the basement membrane of the epithelium)
- Subepithelial or chorional (limited proliferation in the conjunctival chorion)
- Compound (proliferation at the basement membrane and in the chorion)

Conjunctival nevus appears in childhood, is often poorly pigmented initially and then becomes pigmented. Some nevi can remain achromic, and the pigmentation can be heterogeneous.

When pseudocysts are present within the nevus, the nevus is called "Parinaud's epithelial-cystic nevus".

14.1.1 Subepithelial Nevus

This patient (Fig. 14.1) has a pigmented tumor of the temporal bulbar conjunctiva of homogeneous brown colour.

The IVCM features are as follows (Fig. 14.2a–d):

- Absence of disarrangement of the epithelial layers: epithelium (*red stars*) and basement membrane (*green arrows*)
- Hyperreflective homogeneous regularly distributed roundish cells (*yellow stars*) organized in nests (*blue stars*) in the stroma

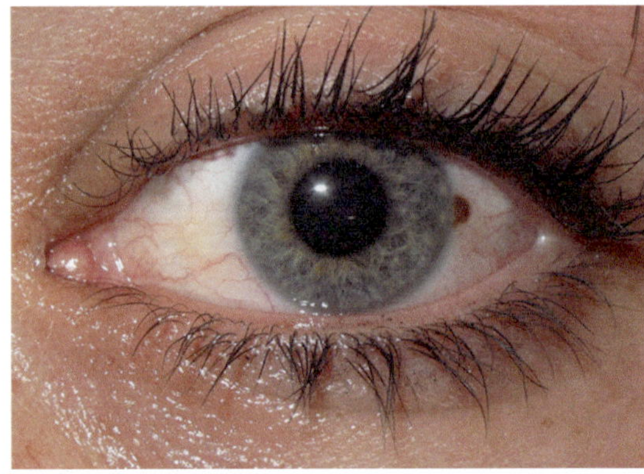

Fig. 14.1 Clinical aspect of subepithelial nevus

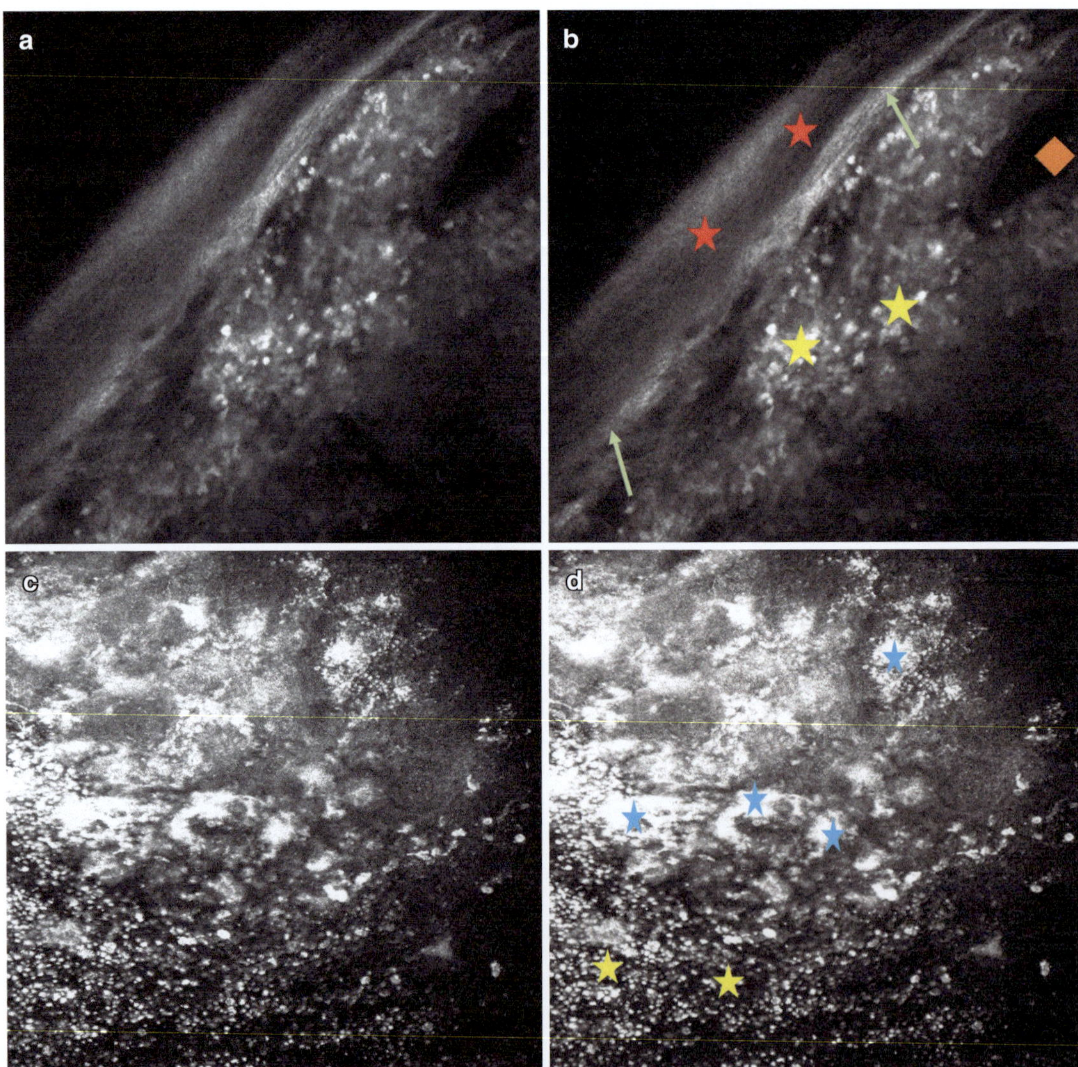

Fig. 14.2 IVCM features of subepithelial nevus (**a**–**d**)

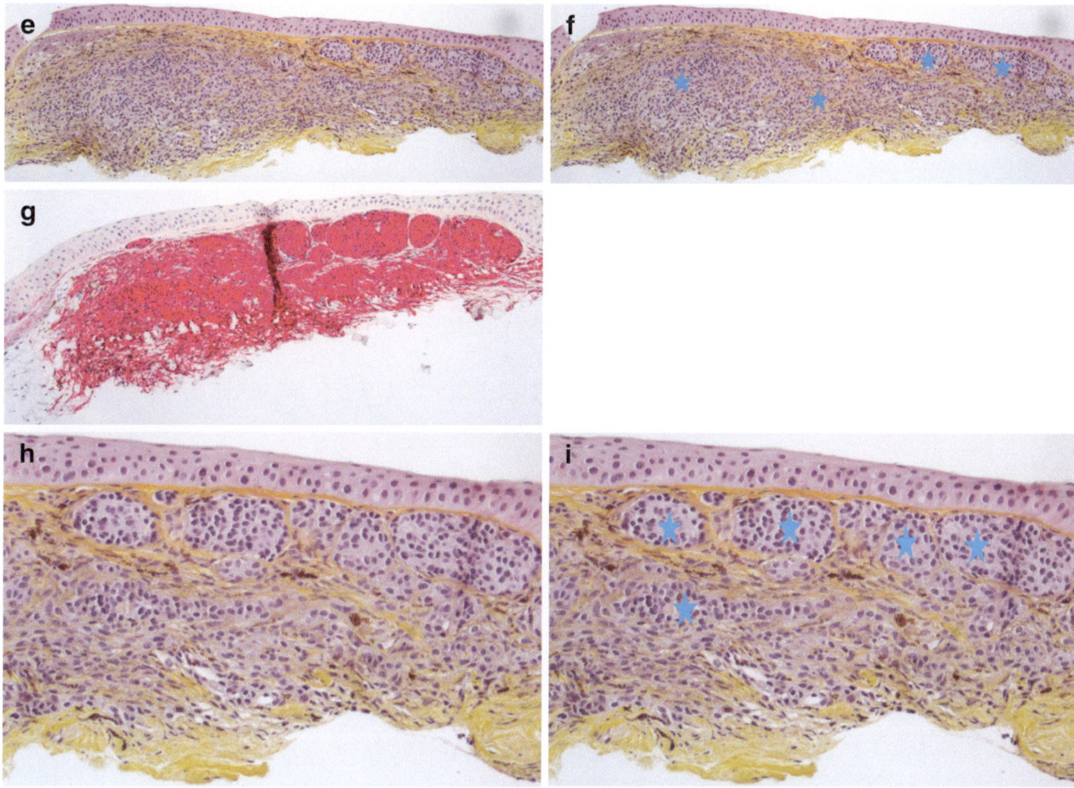

Fig. 14.3 Histological features of subepithelial nevus (**e–i**). (**e, f**) ×100 HES. (**g**) ×100 Anti-Melan-A Ab. (**h, i**) ×200 HES

- Stromal pseudocyst-like structures (*orange diamond*) that can be partly filled with monomorphous material
- Absence of pagetoid cells

On optical microscopy the histologic features are as follows (Fig. 14.3e–i):

- At low magnification (e, f), melanocyte proliferation occurs at the chorion level, in the form of nests (*blue stars*). It stains (in pink) positively for anti-Melan-A antibody (g).
- At high magnification (h, i), no cytonuclear atypia or mitosis is visible.

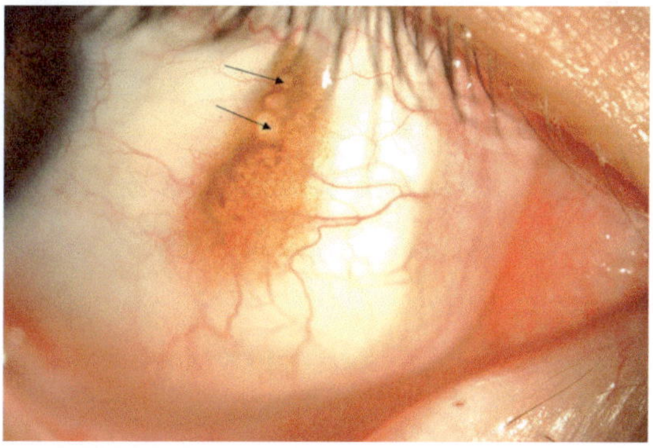

Fig. 14.4 Clinical aspect of junctional nevus: slit-lamp photography

14.1.2 Junctional Nevus

This patient (Fig. 14.4) has a pigmented tumor of the nasal bulbar conjunctiva, which is light brown in color. Cysts are present (*black arrows*).

The IVCM features are as follows (Fig. 14.5a–d):

- Epithelium-chorion junction shows nests of small hyperreflecting roundish cells corresponding to the proliferation of melanocytes (*blue stars*). The cystic structures are non-reflective and round and have a regular wall (*orange diamonds*).

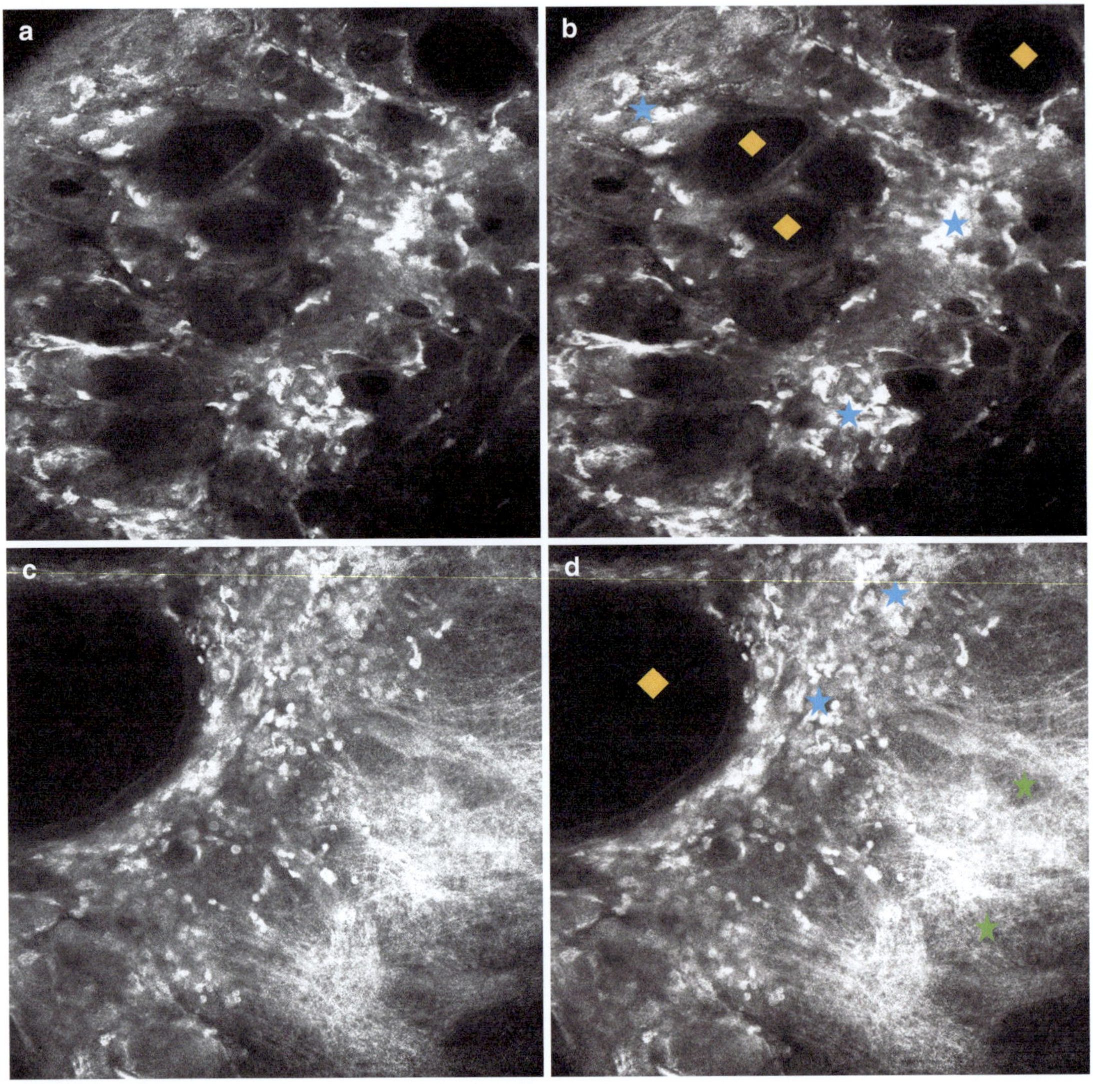

Fig. 14.5 IVCM features of junctional nevus (**a**–**d**)

– Chorion (*green stars*) does not have any hyperreflective roundish cells.

On optical microscopy the histologic features are as follows (Fig. 14.6e–i):

– At low magnification (e–g), melanocyte proliferation is junctional and in the form of nests (*blue stars*). It stains (in pink) positively for anti-Melan-A antibody (g). Cysts (*orange diamonds*) are formed by invagination of the conjunctival epithelium.
– At high magnification (h, i), no cytonuclear atypia or mitosis is visible.

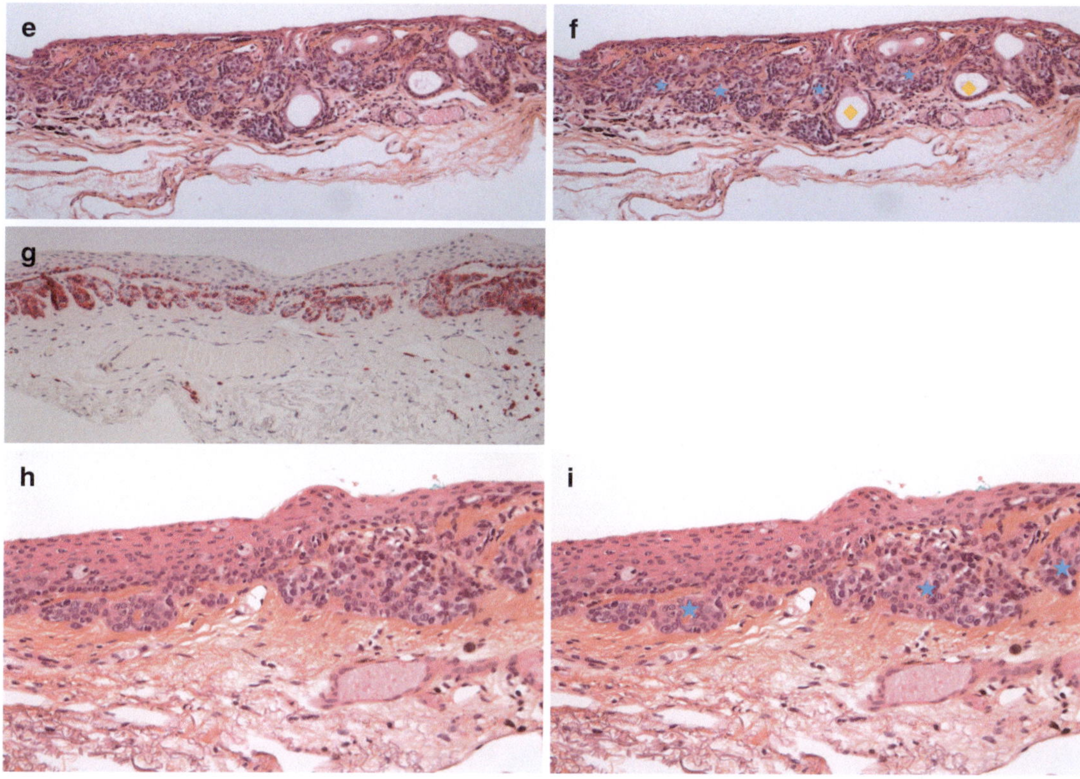

Fig. 14.6 Histological features of junctional nevus (**e–i**). (**e**, **f**) ×100 HES. (**g**) ×100 Anti-Melan-A Ab. (**h**, **i**) ×200 HES

14.1.3 Compound Nevus

This patient (Fig. 14.7) has a pigmented tumor of the nasal bulbar conjunctiva. The pigmentation is more prominent in the centre and lighter at the periphery as in a large part of compound nevi.

The IVCM features are as follows (Fig. 14.8a–d):

- Normal conjunctival epithelium (*red star*).
- Nests of small hyperreflecting roundish cells (*blue stars*) at the epithelium-chorion junction and in the underlying chorion corresponding to the proliferation of melanocytes. Vessels are visible (*orange diamonds*)

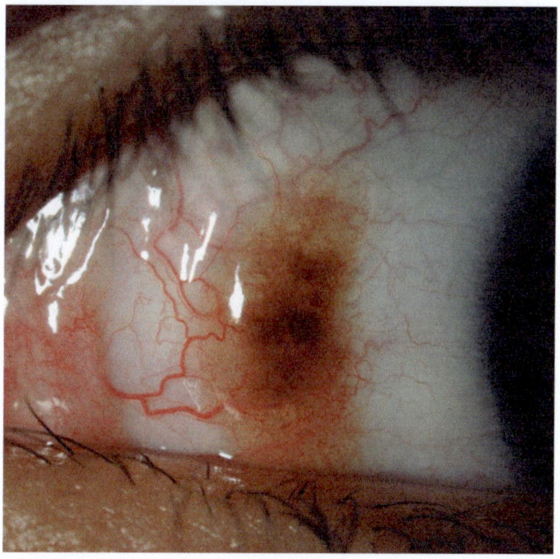

Fig. 14.7 Clinical aspect of compound nevus: slit-lamp photography

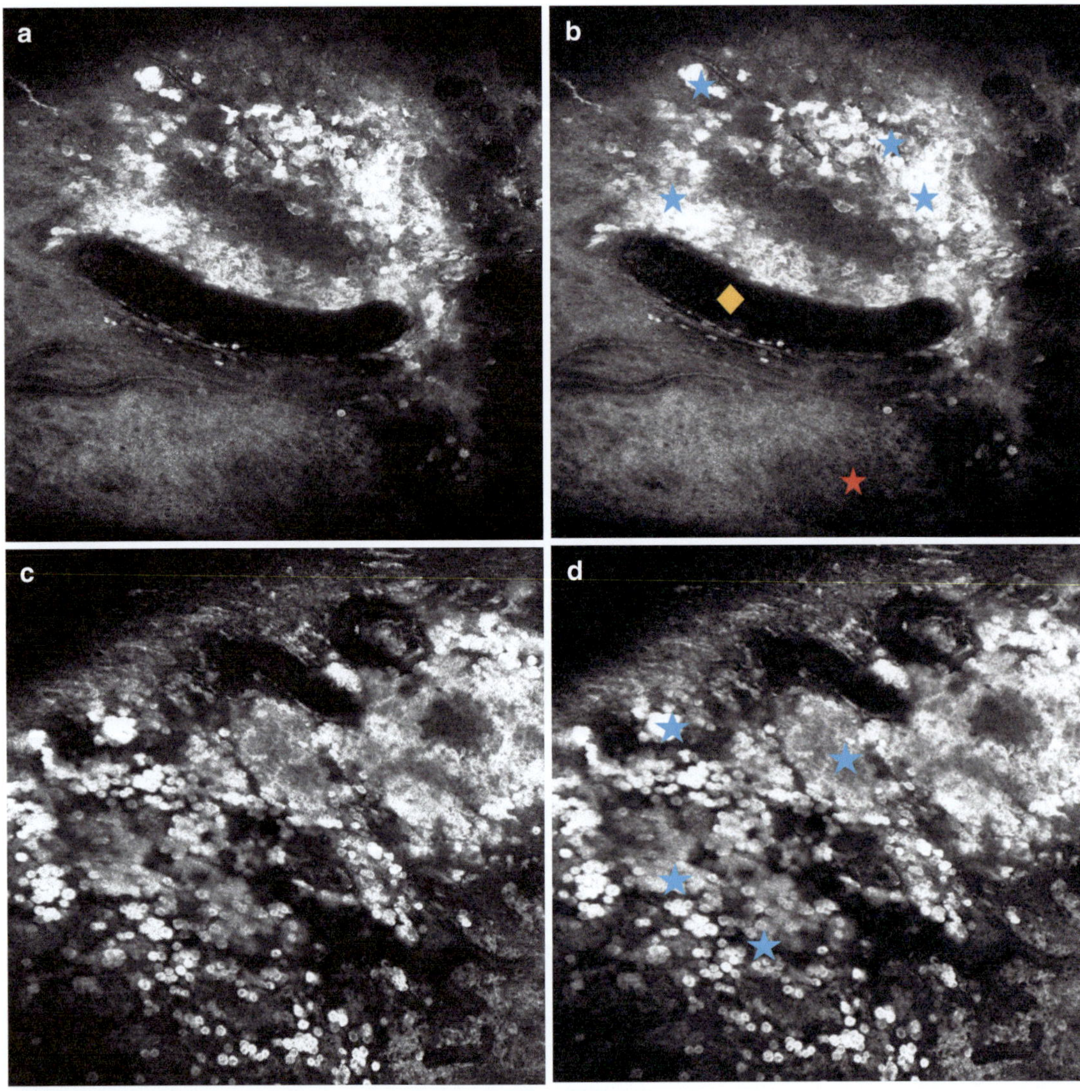

Fig. 14.8 IVCM features of compound nevus (**a**–**d**)

On optical microscopy the histologic features are as follows (Fig. 14.9e–i):

- At low magnification (e–g), melanocyte proliferation is junctional and subepithelial, in the form of nests (*blue stars*). It stains (in pink) positively for anti-Melan-A antibody (g).
- At high magnification (h, i), no cytonuclear atypia or mitosis is visible.

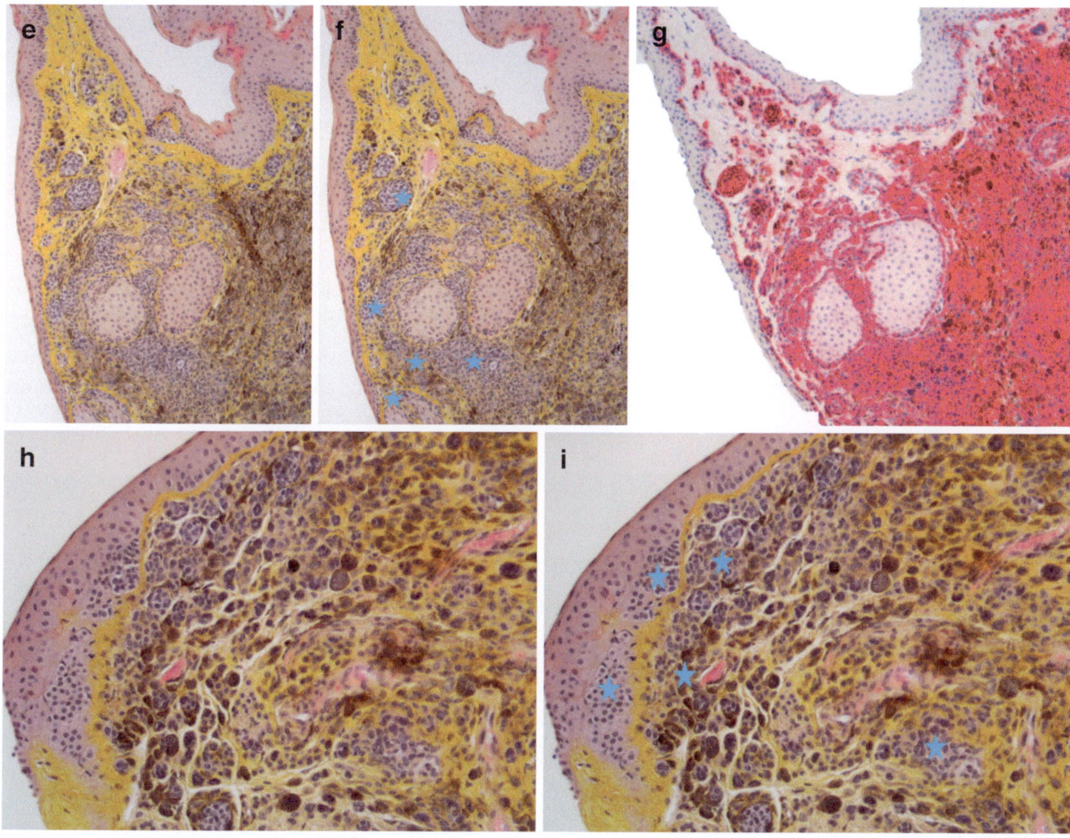

Fig. 14.9 Histological features of compound nevus (**e**–**i**). (**e**, **f**) ×100 HES. (**g**) ×100 Anti-Melan-A Ab. (**h**, **i**) ×200 HES

14.2 Primary Acquired Melanosis (PAM)

14.2.1 Primary Acquired Melanosis Without Atypia

The histological aspect of PAM without atypia and ethnic melanosis (or benign acquired melanosis) is similar. Benign acquired melanosis affects patients with dark phototypes, is bilateral and occurs in the first decades of life, whereas PAM without atypia unilaterally affects older subjects with any phototype.

PAM without atypia (Fig. 14.10) is a homogeneous brown macular pigmentation with irregular contours of the conjunctiva (most often bulbar). PAM without atypia does not contain cysts unlike conjunctival nevus.

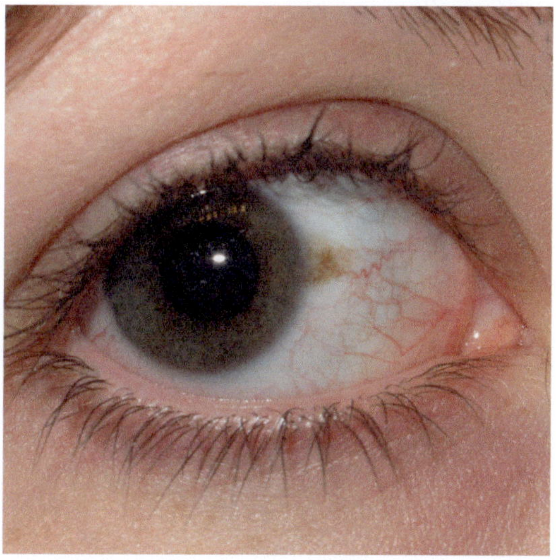

Fig. 14.10 Clinical aspect of primary acquired melanosis without atypia

The IVCM features are as follows (Fig. 14.11a–d):

- Normal conjunctival epithelium with regular honeycomb pattern (not shown here) and possible isolated small pagetoid hyperreflective dendritic cells (not shown here)
- At the conjunctival-chorion epithelium junction, homogeneous small hyperreflective roundish (*red arrows*) and dendritic cells (*yellow circles*) regularly arranged in a single cell layer along the basement membrane of the epithelium and corresponding to a proliferation of melanocytes
- No melanocytes present in the underlying chorion (*green star*)

On optical microscopy the histologic features are as folows (Fig. 14.12e–j):

- At low magnification (e–h), the conjunctival epithelial melanocytic component consists of a continuous lentiginous proliferation of melanocytes without atypia (*blue dotted lines*) and without

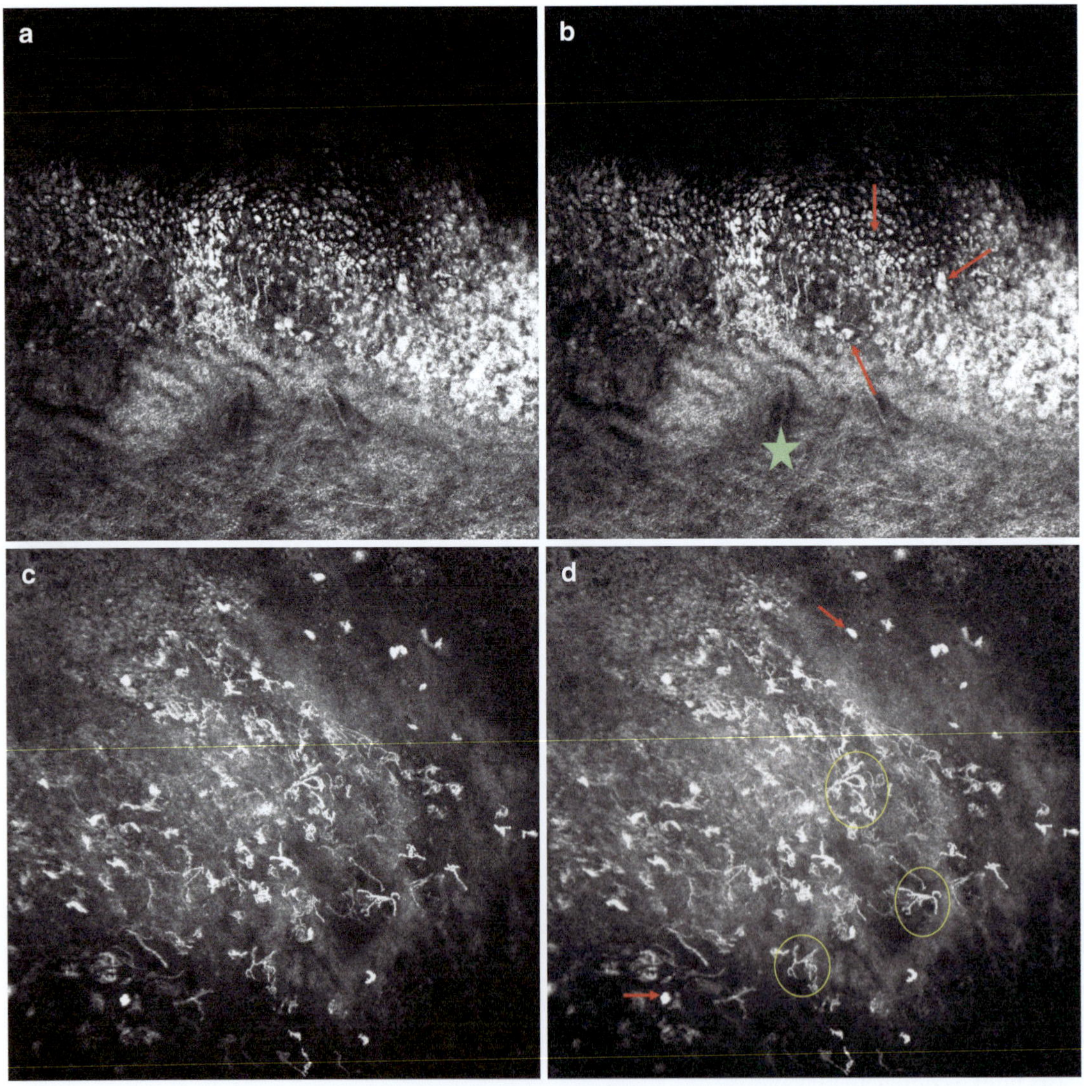

Fig. 14.11 IVCM features of primary acquired melanosis without atypia (**a**–**d**)

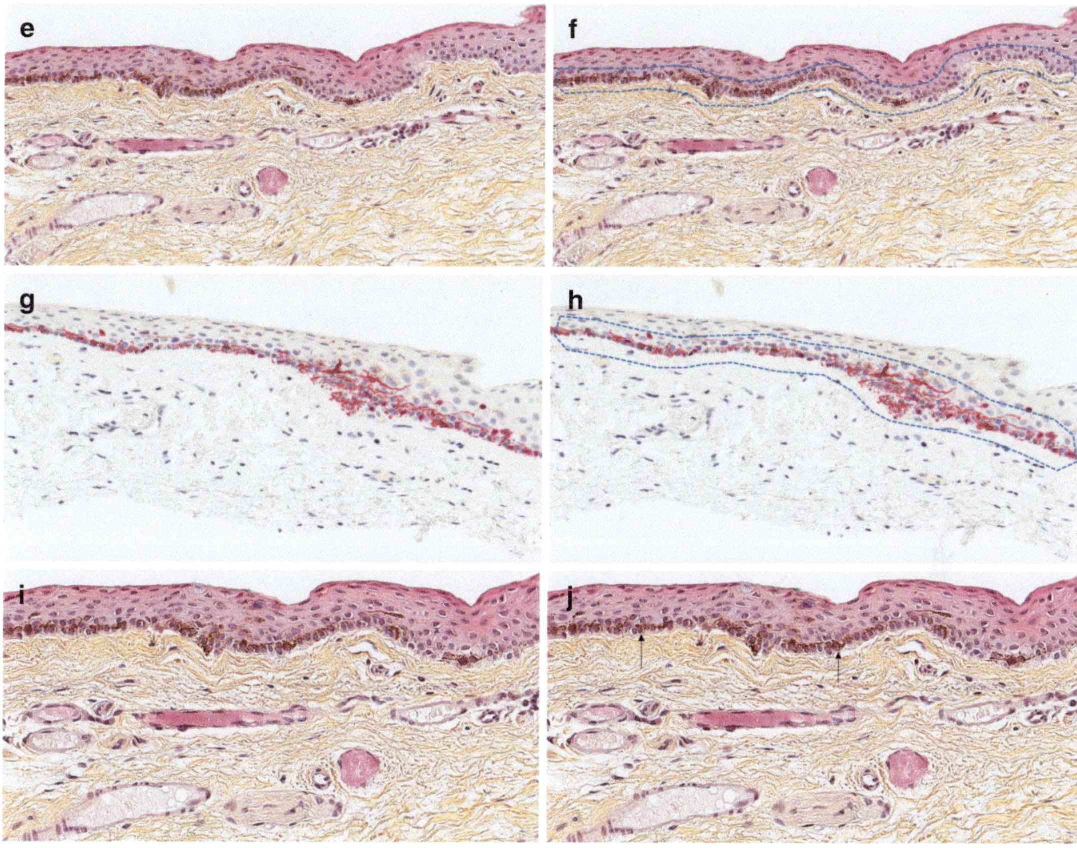

Fig. 14.12 Histological features of primary acquired melanosis without atypia (**e–j**). (**e**, **f**) ×100 HES. (**g**, **h**) ×100 Anti-Melan-A Ab. (**i**, **j**) ×200 HES

extension of the underlying chorion. This proliferation is immunoreactive for Melan-A with cytoplasmic staining (*blue dotted line*).

- At high magnification (i, j), these melanocytes are regular in size and shape, with an eosinophilic cytoplasm, and unevenly overloaded with pigment (*black arrows*). They do not show any image of atypia.

14.2.2 Primary Acquired Melanosis with Atypia

PAM without atypia has no evolutionary potential towards conjunctival melanoma unlike PAM with atypia (progressive risk up to 50%) [1–4].

The clinical aspect (Fig. 14.13) of PAM with atypia is similar to PAM without atypia: it is a

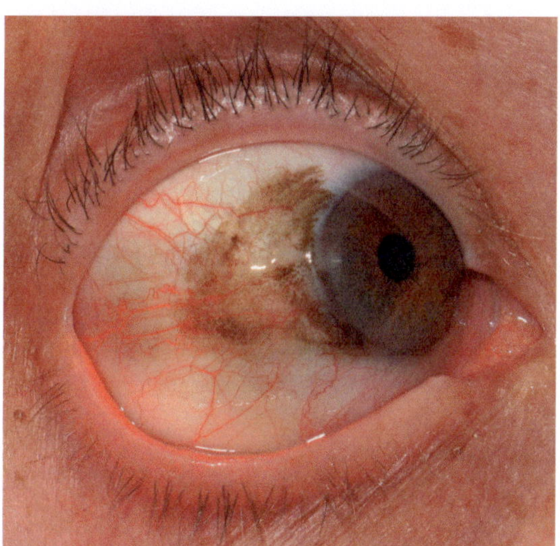

Fig. 14.13 Clinical aspect of primary acquired melanosis with atypia

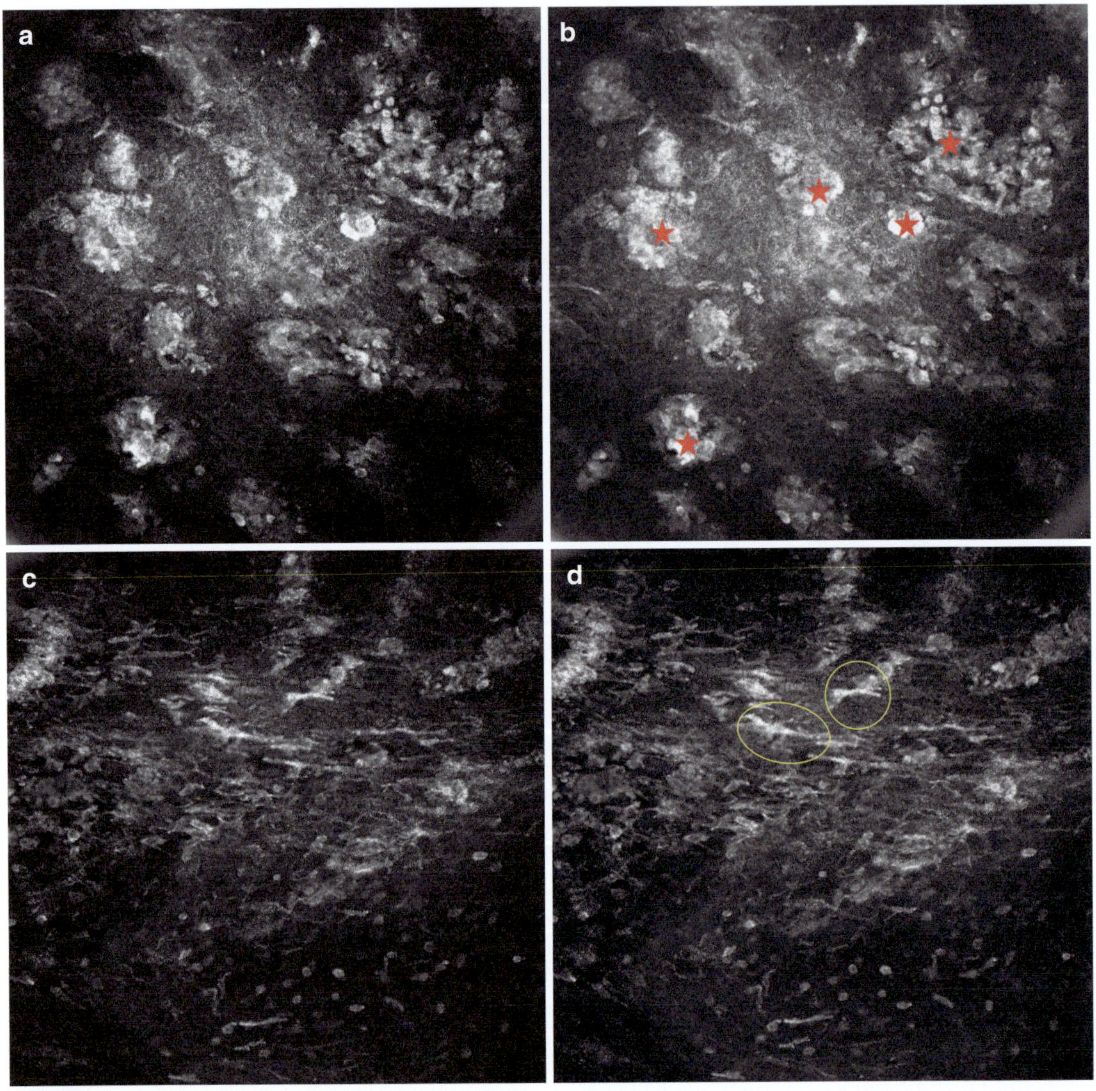

Fig. 14.14 IVCM features of primary acquired melanosis with atypia (**a**–**d**)

brown macular pigmentation of the conjunctiva (most often bulbar) with irregular contours. PAM with atypia may have heterogeneous pigmentation, and changes may occur over time (pigment modification or growth).

The IVCM features are as follows (Fig. 14.14a–d):

- Irregular melanocytes throughout the epithelium without crossing the basement membrane of the epithelium in the form of large hyperreflective roundish (*red stars*) or dendritic (*yellow circles*) cells grouped into clusters or isolated

On optical microscopy the histologic features are as follows (Fig. 14.15e–i):

- At low magnification (e–g), the conjunctival epithelial melanocytic component consists of a junctional proliferation (intraepithelial) (*blue dotted lines*) with clusters of cells (*red stars*). This proliferation is immunoreactive for Melan-A with cytoplasmic staining (g).
- At high magnification (h, i), melanocytes have an ovoid nucleus with sometimes visible nucleolus (*black arrow*).

Atypia of PAM is histologically classified as minimal, moderate and severe. PAMs with severe

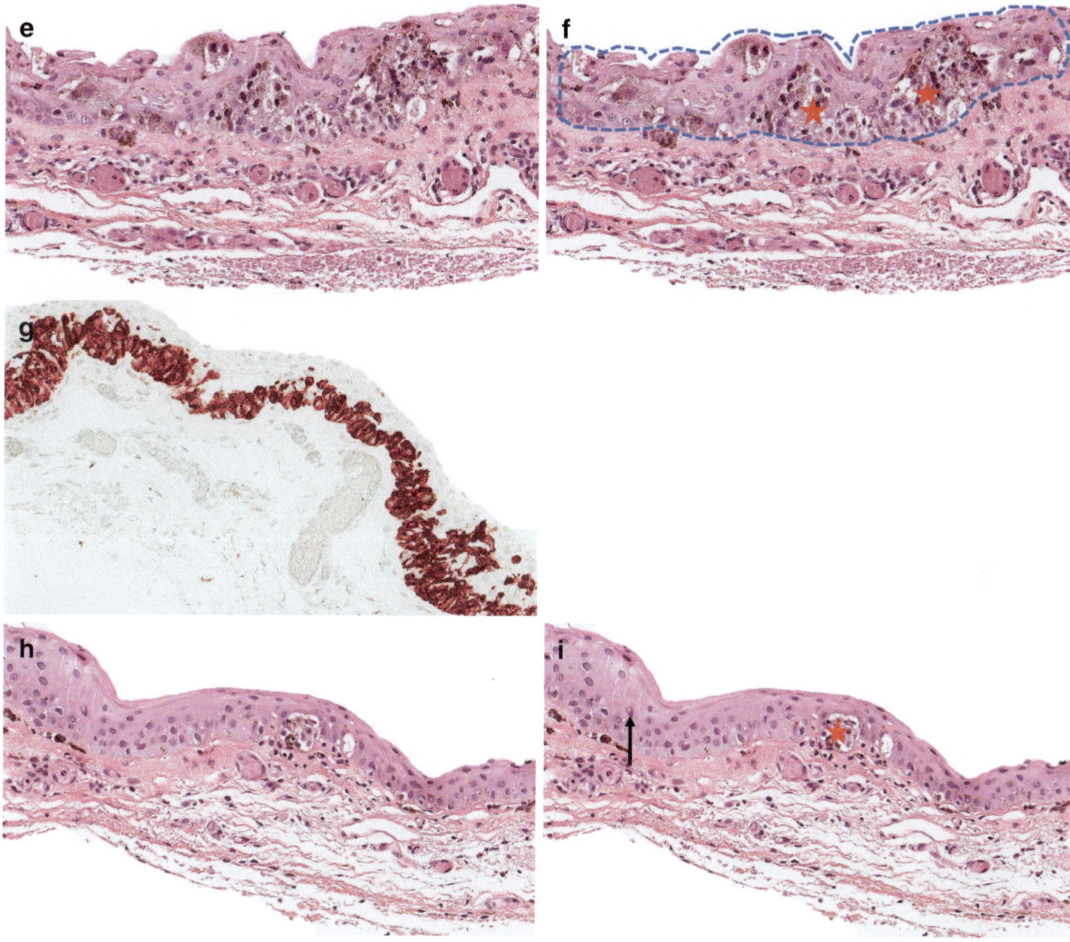

Fig. 14.15 Histological features of primary acquired melanosis with atypia (**e**–**i**). (**e**, **f**) ×100 HES. (**g**) ×100 Anti-Melan-A Ab. (**h**, **i**) ×200 HES

atypia is comparable to in situ conjunctival melanoma and should be treated as such.

14.3 Melanoma

Seventy-four percent of conjunctival melanomas developed from PAM with atypia [1, 5]. Conjunctival melanoma can be pigmented or achromic.

The clinical aspect (Fig. 14.16) of this conjunctival melanoma is a heterogeneous pigmentation of the bulbar conjunctiva with irregular contours. This pigmented tumor has undergone recent changes in pigmentation and size.

The IVCM features are as follows (Fig. 14.17a–e):

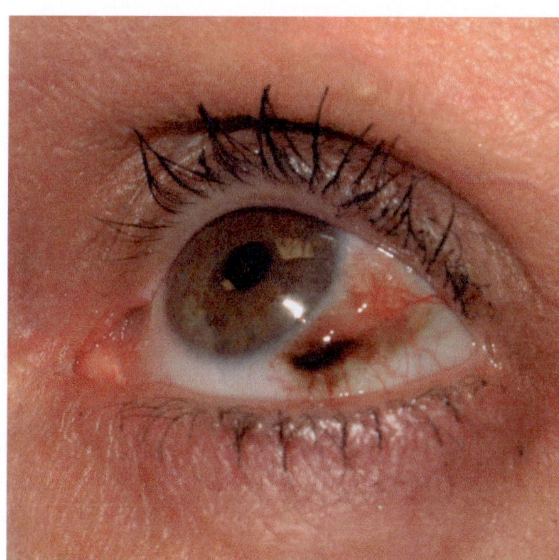

Fig. 14.16 Clinical aspect of conjunctival melanoma

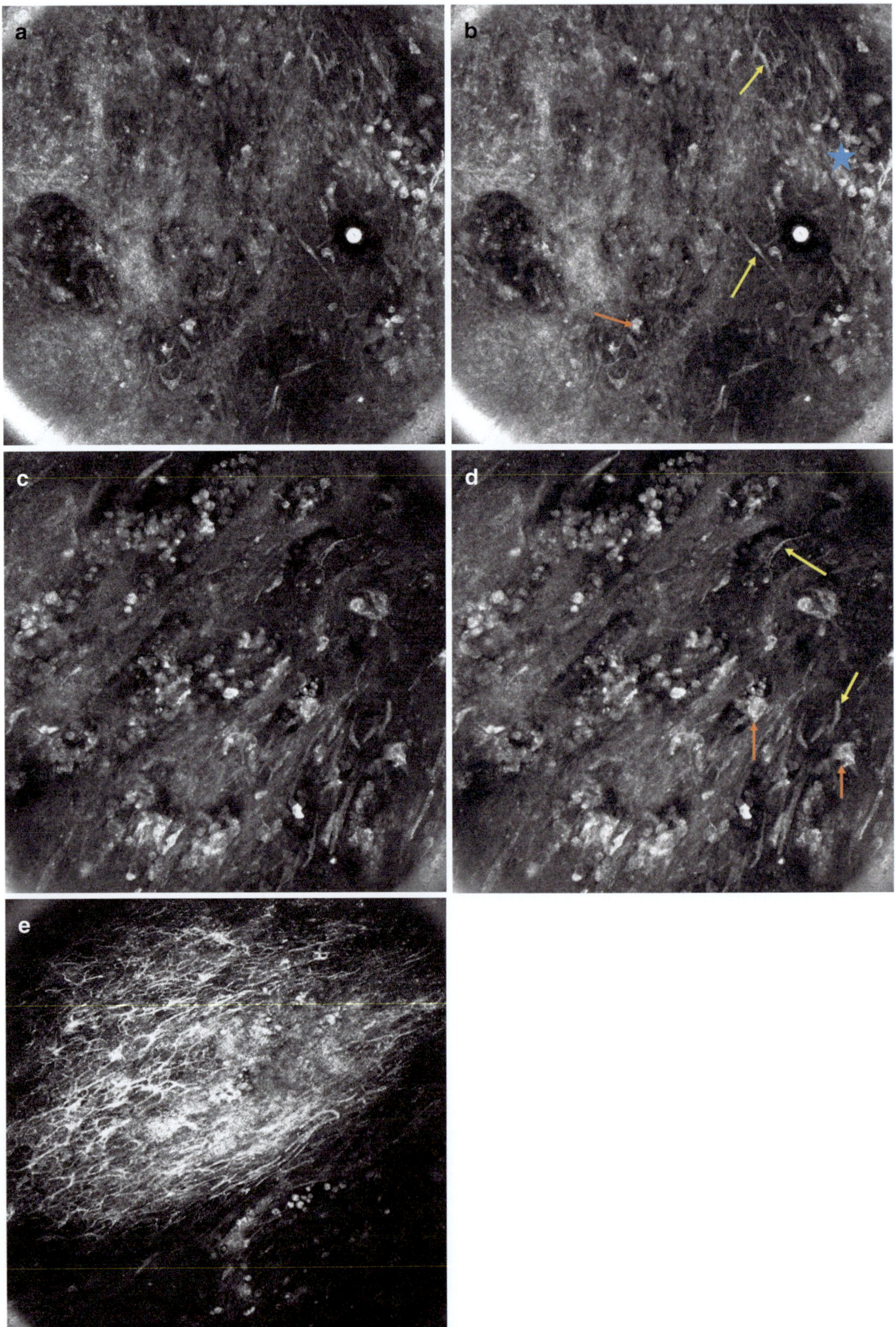

Fig. 14.17 IVCM features of conjunctival melanoma (**a**–**e**)

- Irregular hyperreflective cells of different sizes (usually larger than epithelial cells) and shapes: round (*blue stars*), polygonal (*orange arrows*) and dendritic/fusiform (*yellow arrows, and picture e*) in the epithelium (a, b) and in the stroma (c–e).

Notably, malignant melanocytes have an irregular dendritic shape and their different shape under IVCM is due to the level of their virtual section by IVCM: if they are sectioned at the level of the cellular body they appear as roundish, if they are sectioned at the level of their dendrites they are dendritic/fusiform and if they are sectioned slantwise they can show a polygonal shape.

On optical microscopy the histologic features are as follows (Fig. 14.18f–j):

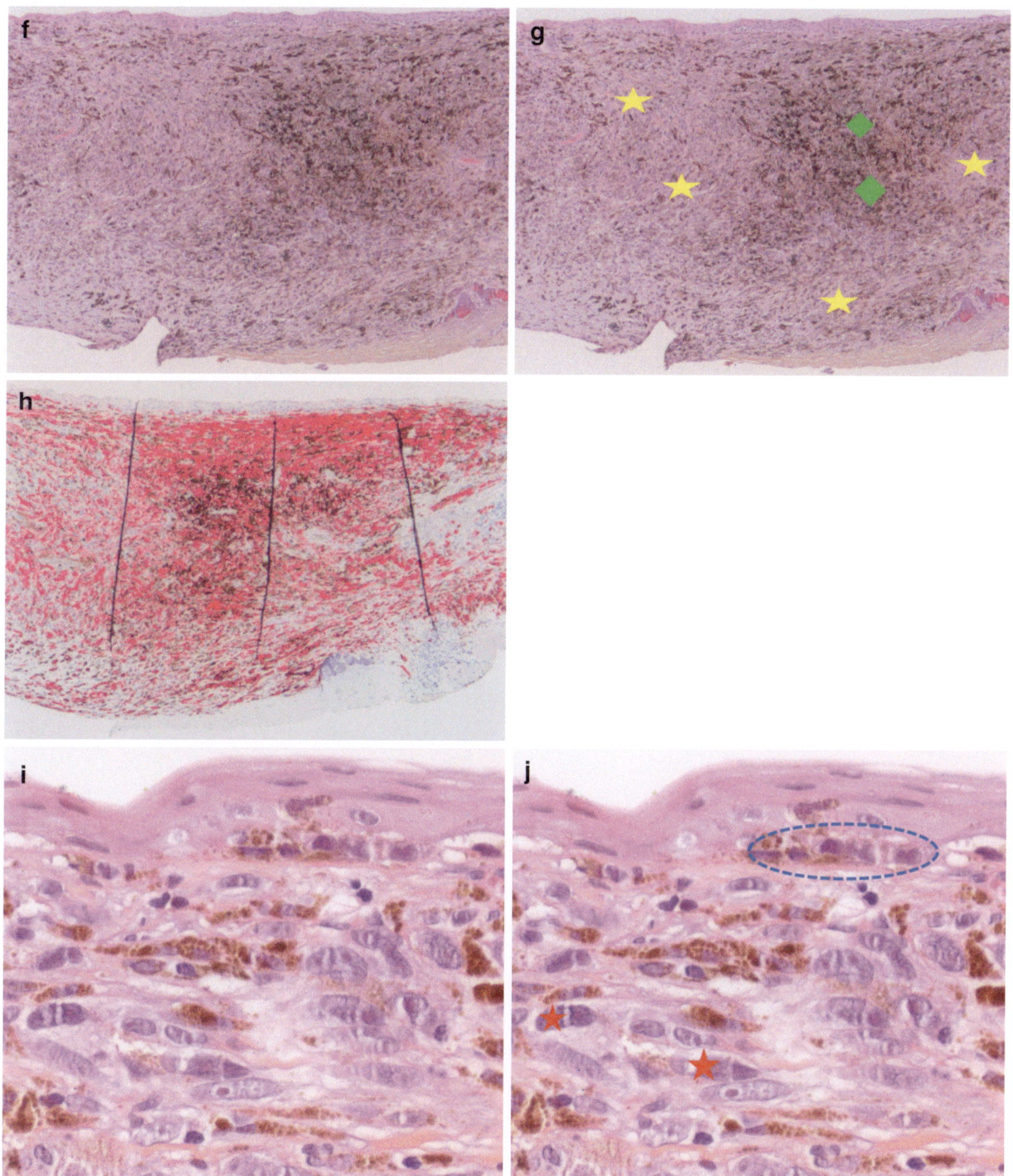

Fig. 14.18 Histological features of conjunctival melanoma (**f–j**). (**f, g**) ×50 HES. (**h**) ×50 Anti-Melan-A Ab. (**i, j**) ×400 HES

- At low magnification (f–h), melanocyte proliferation (*yellow stars*) of pleomorphic melanocytes is seen, sometimes fusiform in the epithelium and the stroma. The cytoplasm of the cells is overloaded with pigment (*green diamonds*). This proliferation is immunoreactive for Melan-A for cytoplasmic staining (h).
- At high magnification (i, j), melanocytes, mostly fusiform (*red stars*), have dysmorphic nuclei, with an unevenly condensed chromatin. In this case, the intraepithelial melanocytic component consists of a lentiginous proliferation (*blue dotted line*).

References

1. Kao A, Afshar A, Bloomer M, Damato B. Management of primary acquired melanosis, nevus, and conjunctival melanoma. Cancer Control. 2016;23:117–25.
2. Farber M, Schutzer P, Mihm MC. Pigmented lesions of the conjunctiva. J Am Acad Dermatol. 1998;38:971–8.
3. Shields CL, Shields JA. Tumors of the conjunctiva and cornea. Surv Ophthalmol. 2004;49:3–24.
4. Novais GA, Fernandes BF, Belfort RN, Castiglione E, Cheema DP, Burnier MN. Incidence of melanocytic lesions of the conjunctiva in a review of 10,675 ophthalmic specimens. Int J Surg Pathol. 2010;18:60–3.
5. Shields CL, Chien JL, Surakiatchanukul T, Sioufi K, Lally SE, Shields JA. Conjunctival tumors: review of clinical features, risks, biomarkers, and outcomes – the 2017. J Ophthalmol. 2017;6:109–20.

Non-epithelial and Non-melanocytic Conjunctival Tumors

15

Thibaud Garcin, Mathilde Kaspi, Cyril Habougit, Damien Grivet, Jean-Luc Perrot, and Elisa Cinotti

Contents

Abbreviations

Ab	Antibodies
HES	Hematoxylin-eosin-saffron stain
IVCM	In vivo reflectance confocal microscopy
MALT	Mucosa-associated lymphoid tissue

T. Garcin (✉) · M. Kaspi · D. Grivet
Department of Ophthalmology, University Hospital of Saint-Etienne, Saint-Etienne, France
e-mail: garcinthibaud@gmail.com; mathilde.kaspi@gmail.com; damien.grivet@chu-st-etienne.fr

C. Habougit
Department of Pathology, University Hospital of Saint-Etienne, Saint-Etienne, France
e-mail: cyril.habougit@chu-st-etienne.fr

J.-L. Perrot
Department of Dermatology, University Hospital of Saint-Etienne, Saint-Etienne, France
e-mail: j.luc.perrot@chu-st-etienne.fr

E. Cinotti
Department of Dermatology, University of Siena, S. Maria alle Scotte Hospital, Siena, Italy
e-mail: elisa.cinotti@unisi.it

15.1 Conjunctival Stroma Degeneration

15.1.1 Pterygium

This patient (Fig. 15.1) has two pterygium. The one in the temporal topography is more severe.

Pterygium is a triangular conjunctivo-corneal lesion with a conjunctival base, translucent at the

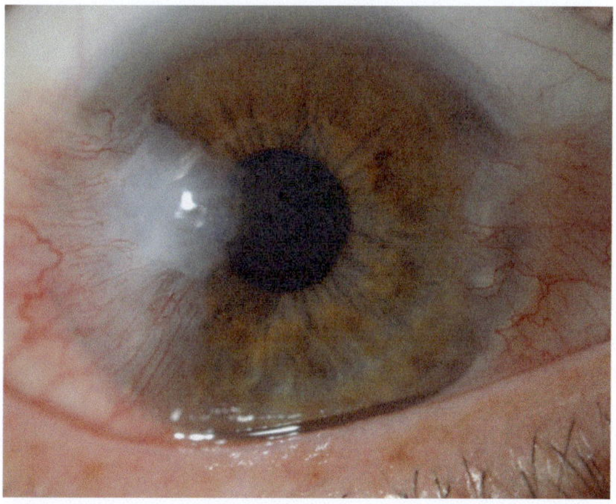

Fig. 15.1 Clinical aspect of pterygium: slit-lamp photography

© Springer Nature Switzerland AG 2020
M. Kaspi et al. (eds.), *Eyelid and Conjunctival Tumors*,
https://doi.org/10.1007/978-3-030-36606-3_15

conjunctival level and gelatinous at the corneal level. Vessels are visible on its surface.

The IVCM features are as follows (Fig. 15.2a–d):

- Fibrovascular proliferation in the chorion (*green diamonds*) is well demarcated from the corneal epithelium (*blue stars*). Some large vessels are visible (*yellow arrow*).
- Normal conjunctival epithelium is seen (not shown here).
- Possible increased leukocytes (small, hyperreflective, roundish homogeneous cells) in the stroma are visible.

On optical microscopy the histologic features are as follows (Fig. 15.3e–h):

- At low magnification (e, f), in this case the fibrovascular proliferation is lobular in architecture with a finger pocket shape (*black star*). Hematologic slicks are visible (*green diamonds*).
- At high magnification (g, h), conjunctival epithelium is thickened and contains an increased number of goblet cells (*orange arrow*). Goblet cells are characterized by a dilated apical pole and a foamy cytoplasm slightly stained due to the synthesis and accumulation of substances

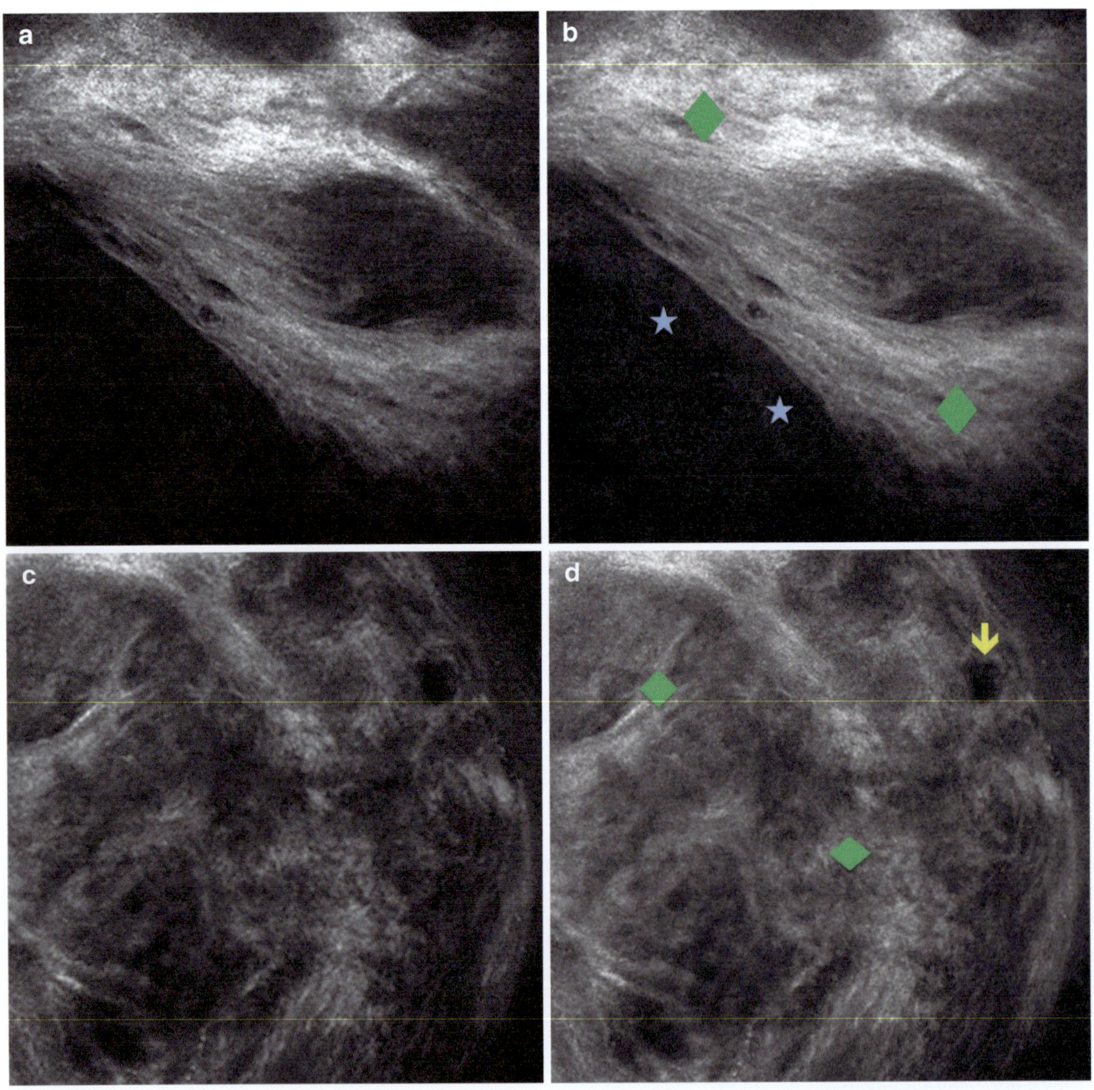

Fig. 15.2 IVCM features of pterygium (**a–d**)

rich in glycosaminoglycan. They are found in normal conjunctival epithelium and are increased in number in pterygium, possibly as a consequence of the exposure of the anterior segment of the eye to irritant agents. Although in this case the epithelium is thickened, pterygium can have a hyperplastic or thinned epithelium. In the chorion, the connective tissue is densified and highly vascularized (*yellow arrows*). Some collagen bundles have a degenerative aspect (*green circle*).

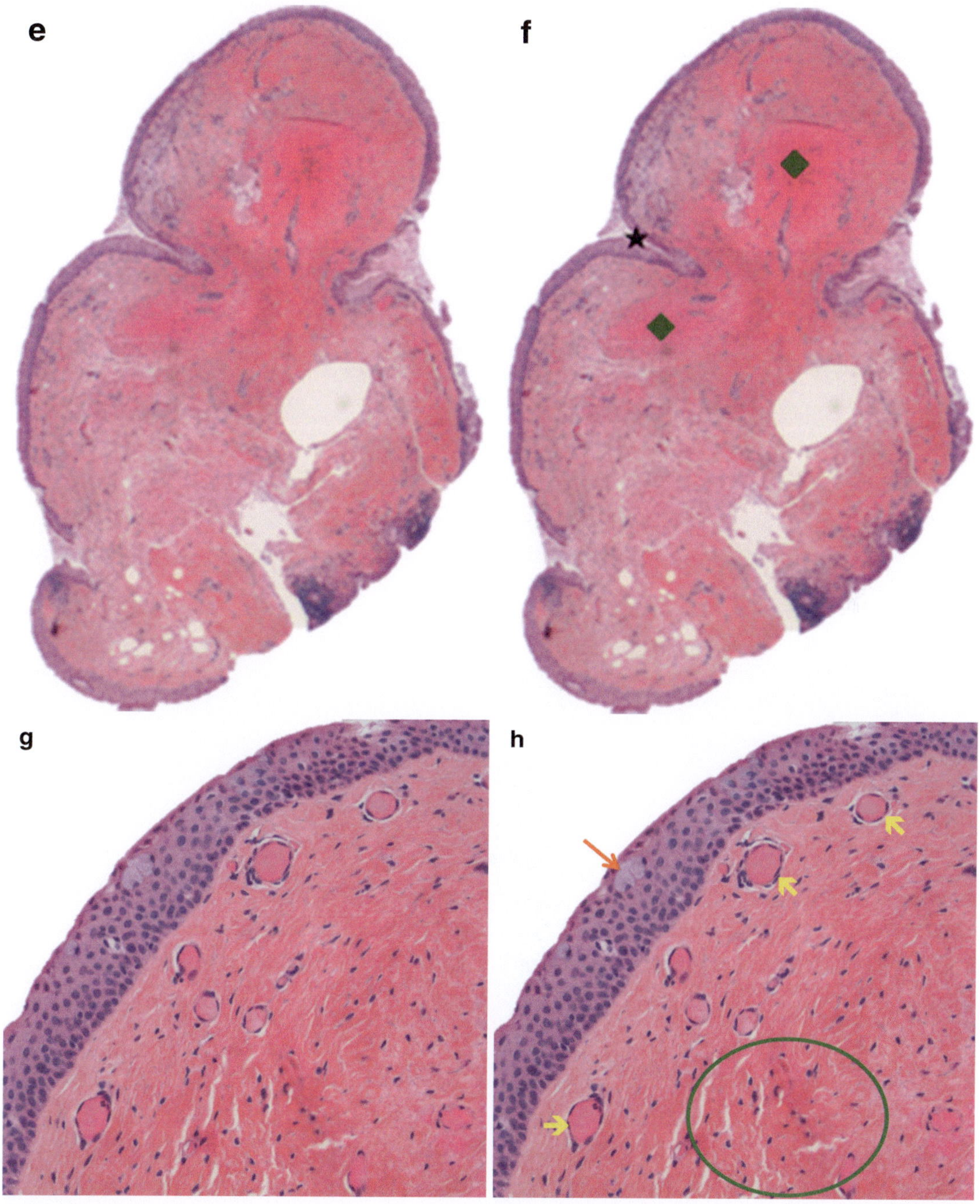

Fig. 15.3 Histological features of pterygium (**e-h**). (**e**, **f**) ×25 HES. (**g**, **h**) ×200 HES

15.1.2 Pinguecula

Pinguecula (Fig. 15.4) is a triangular yellowish conjunctival lesion with an external base. Pinguecula does not grow onto the corneal surface.

The IVCM features are as follows (Fig. 15.5a–d):

- Regular conjunctival epithelium (*red stars*): in pinguecula the epithelium can be thinned or hyperplastic.
- Clusters of degenerated stroma are visible as hyperreflective homogeneous areas (*orange stars*).

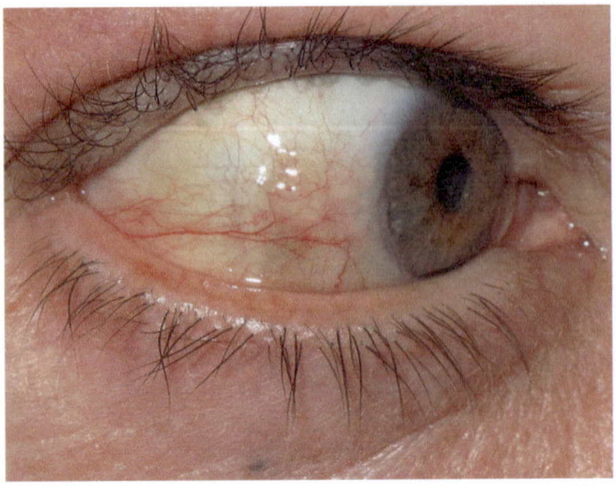

Fig. 15.4 Clinical aspect of pinguecula

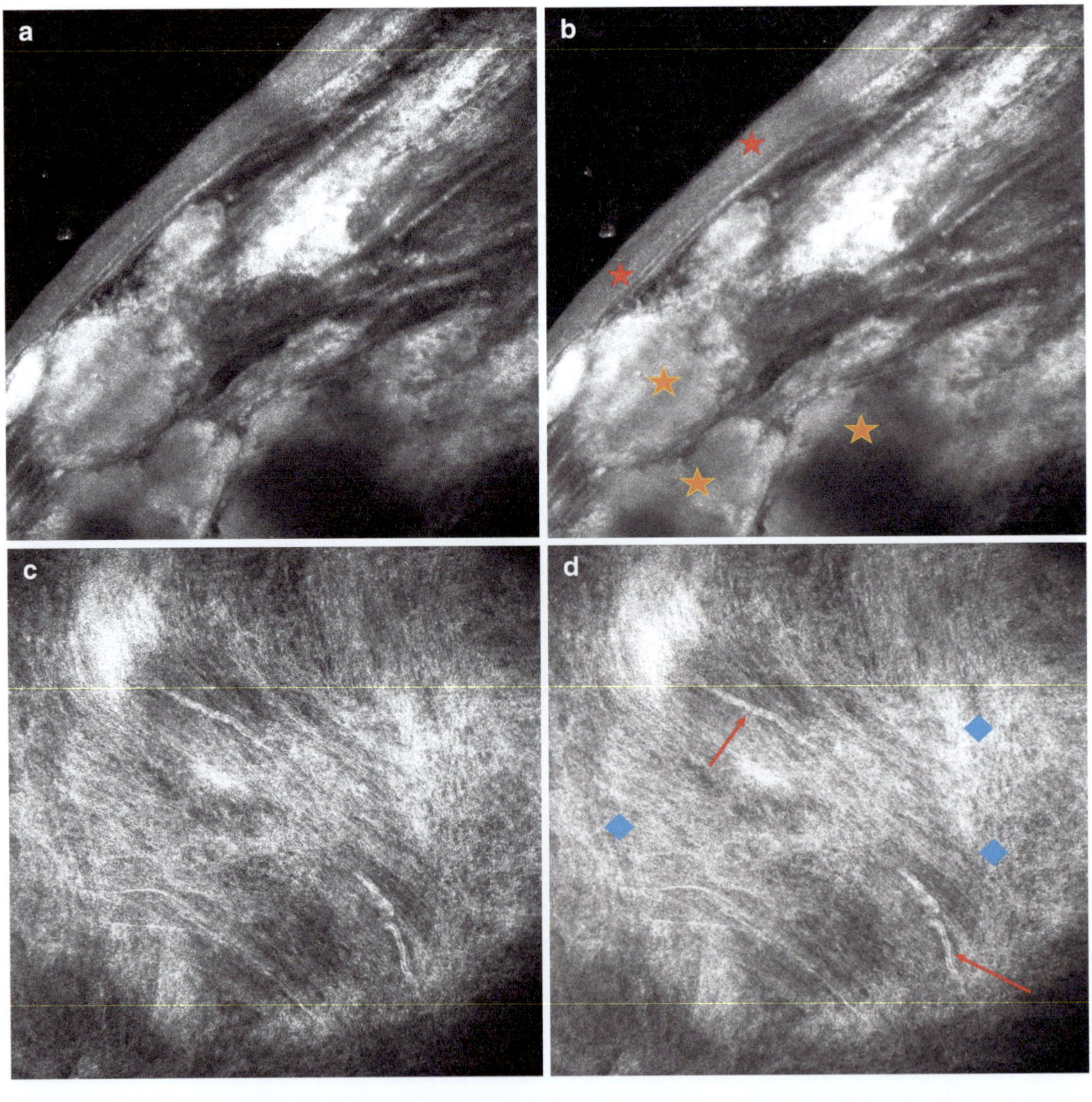

Fig. 15.5 IVCM features of pinguecula (**a**–**d**)

- Fibrous stroma (*blue diamonds*) with degenerated elastic and collagen fibers is presented with a coiled shape (*red arrows*).
- There are no dysplastic epithelial cells.
- Possible increased leukocytes (small, hyperreflective, roundish homogeneous cells) in the stroma.

On optical microscopy the histologic features are as follows (Fig. 15.6e–h):

- At low magnification (e, f), fibrovascular proliferation with a lobular architecture is seen. Hematologic slicks are visible (*green diamonds*).
- At high magnification (g, h), under the epithelium, the connective tissue is densified (*orange stars*) and very vascularized (*yellow arrows*). At greater depth, some collagen bundles have a degenerative aspect (*blue diamonds*).

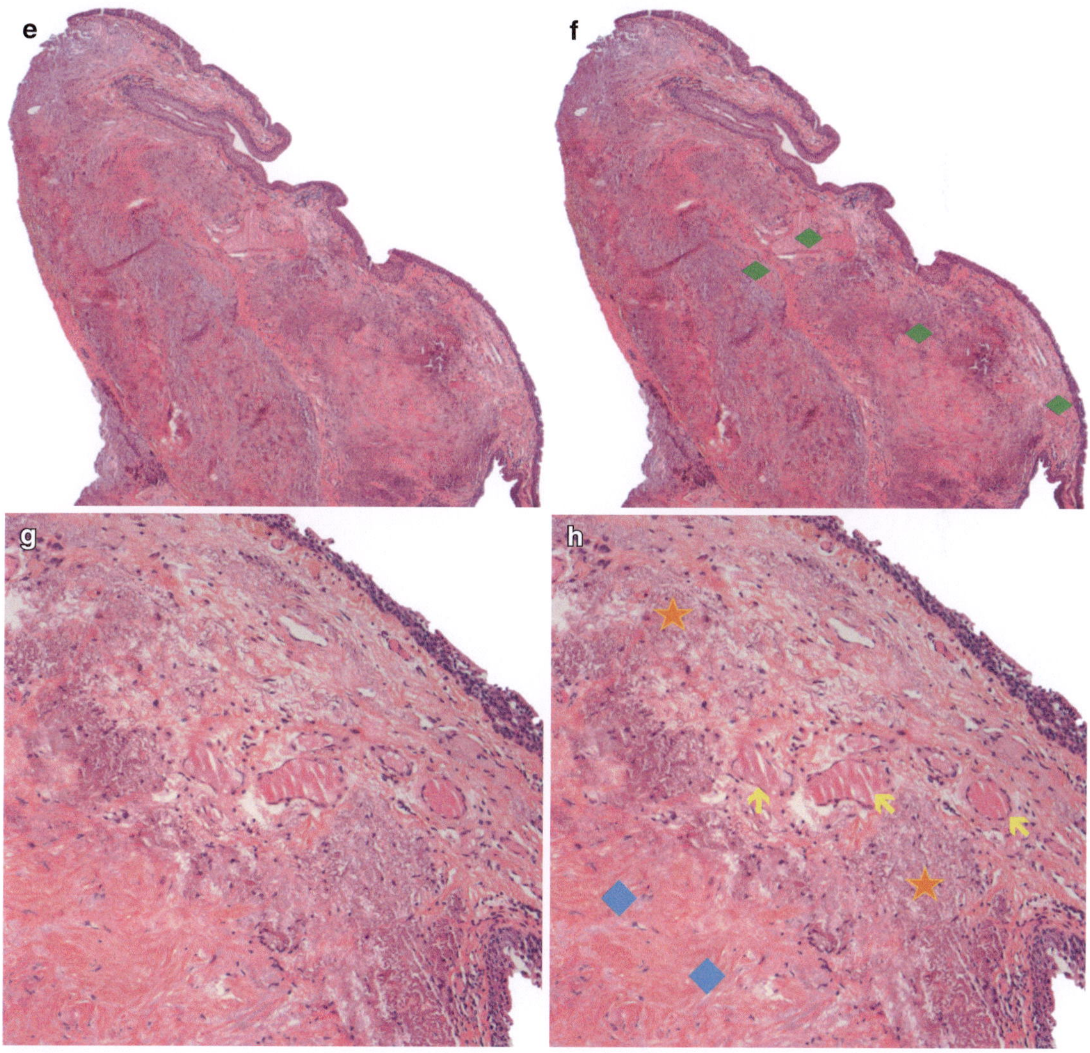

Fig. 15.6 Histological features of pinguecula (**e**–**h**). (**e**, **f**) ×25 HES. (**g**, **h**) ×100 HES

15.2 Lymphoma: B-Cell Lymphoma

15.2.1 Mantle Cell Lymphoma

This patient (Fig. 15.7) has a rapidly growing (for 1 month) plaque of the conjunctival fornix with soft texture and smooth surface.

The IVCM features are as follows (Fig. 15.8a–d):

- Widespread small hyperreflective roundish cells, corresponding to tumor lymphocytes in the chorion (*yellow diamonds and orange stars*)
- Dilated vessels (*green arrows*)

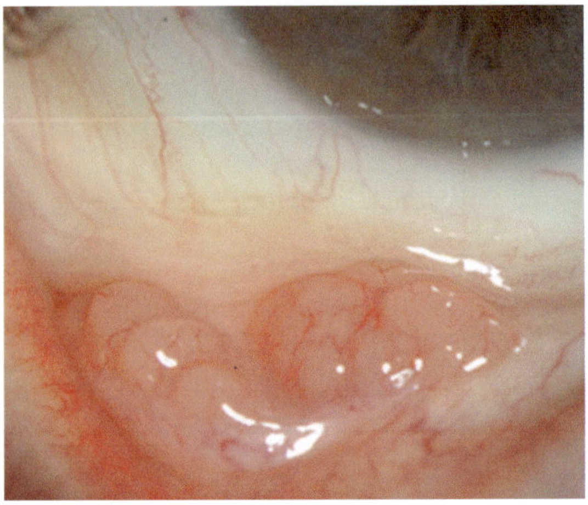

Fig. 15.7 Clinical aspect of B-cell lymphoma

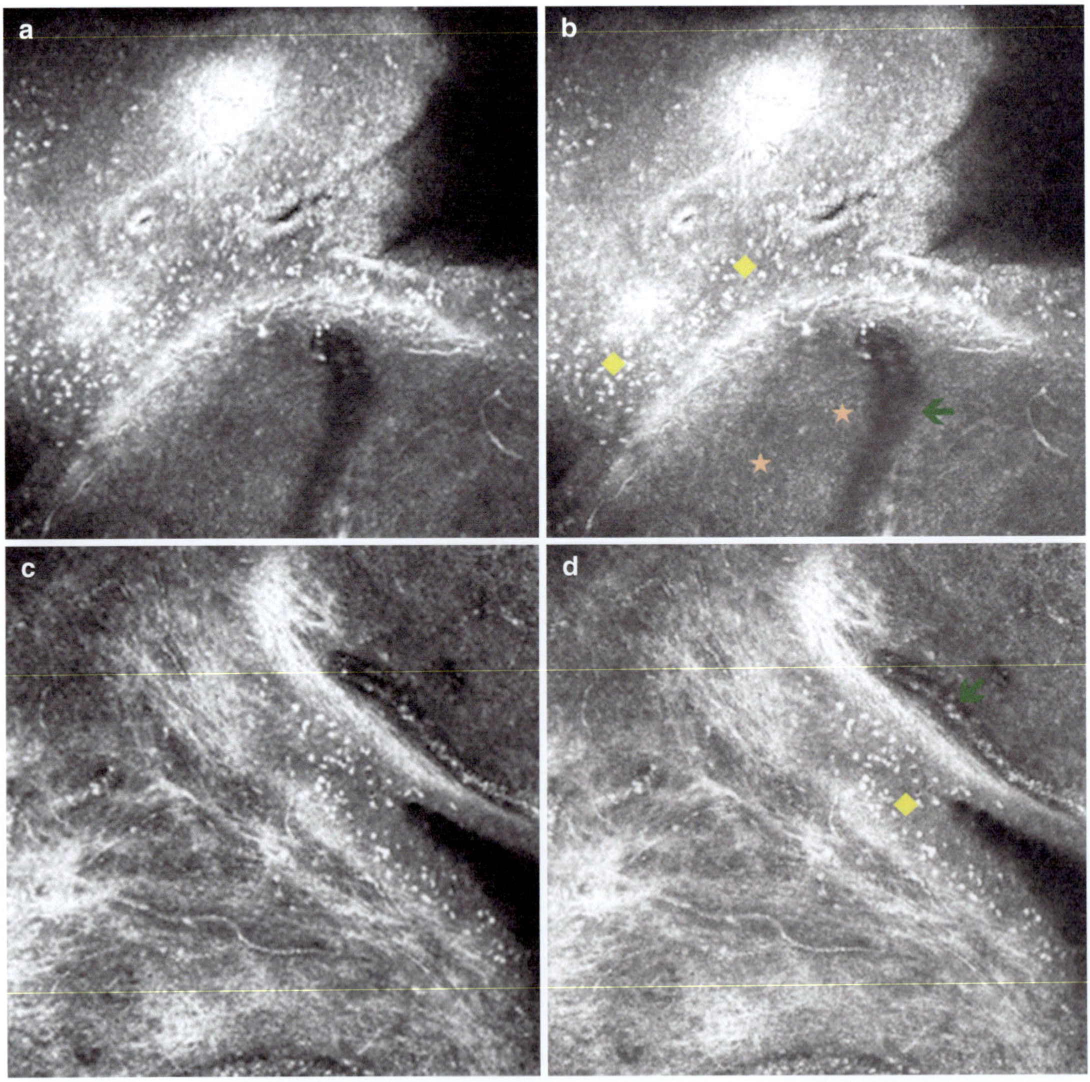

Fig. 15.8 IVCM features of B-cell lymphoma (**a**–**d**)

On optical microscopy the histologic features are as follows (Fig. 15.9e–i):

- At low magnification (e, f), there is proliferation of small monomorphic lymphocytes in the chorion (*orange stars*).
- Immunohistochemistry (g) shows that this proliferation is marked by the anti-CD20 antibody in brown (g.1) and by the anti-cycline D1 antibody in blue (g.2). Anti-CD5 and anti-CD79a antibody are also positive. In addition,

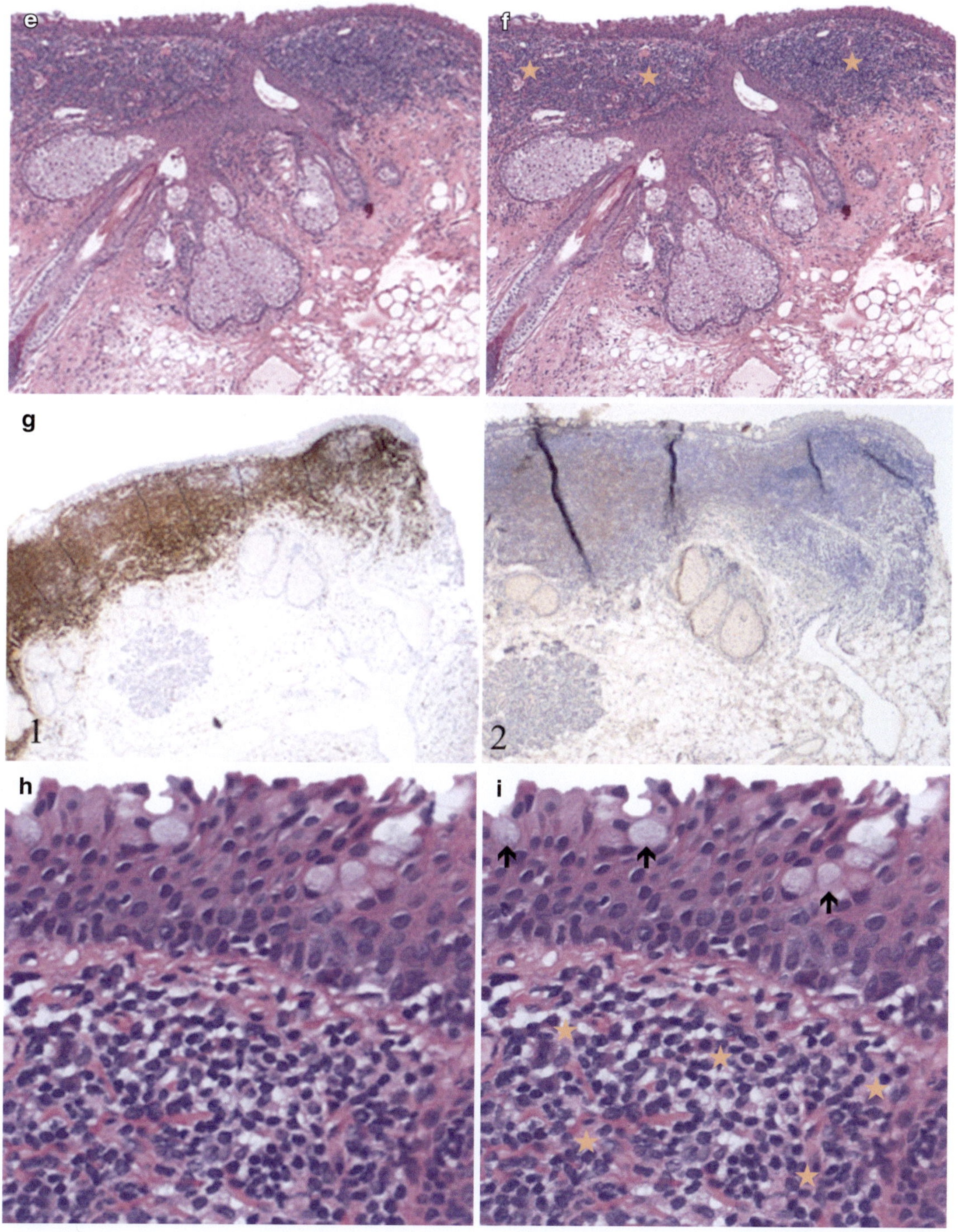

Fig. 15.9 Histological features of B-cell lymphoma (**e**–**i**). (**e**, **f**) ×50 HES. (**g**) ×25 Anti-CD20 Ab (**g**.1), anti-cycline D1 Ab (**g**.2). (**h**, **i**) ×200 HES

there is no immunoreactivity to antibodies against CD3, CD10, and CD23.

– At high magnification (h, i), the architecture is in clusters and composed of small- to medium-sized lymphocytes (*orange stars*). No mitotic figures are observed. The conjunctival epithelium contains goblet cells (*black arrows*).

15.2.2 Mucosa-Associated Lymphoid Tissue (MALT)

MALT (Fig. 15.10) usually presents with a flat or raised salmon-colored conjunctival lesion.

The IVCM features are as follows (Fig. 15.11a–d):

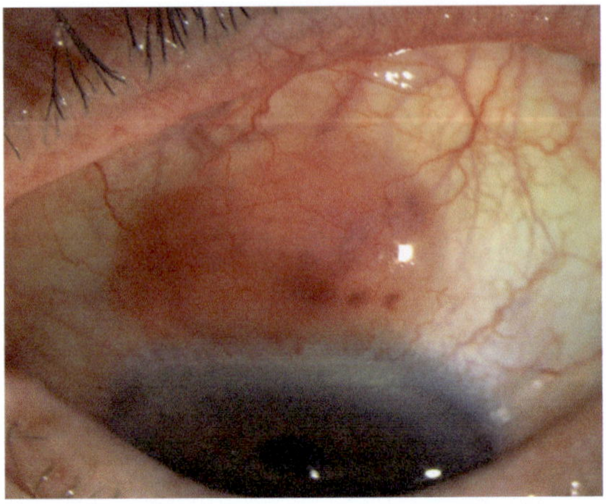

Fig. 15.10 Clinical aspect of mucosa-associated lymphoid tissue

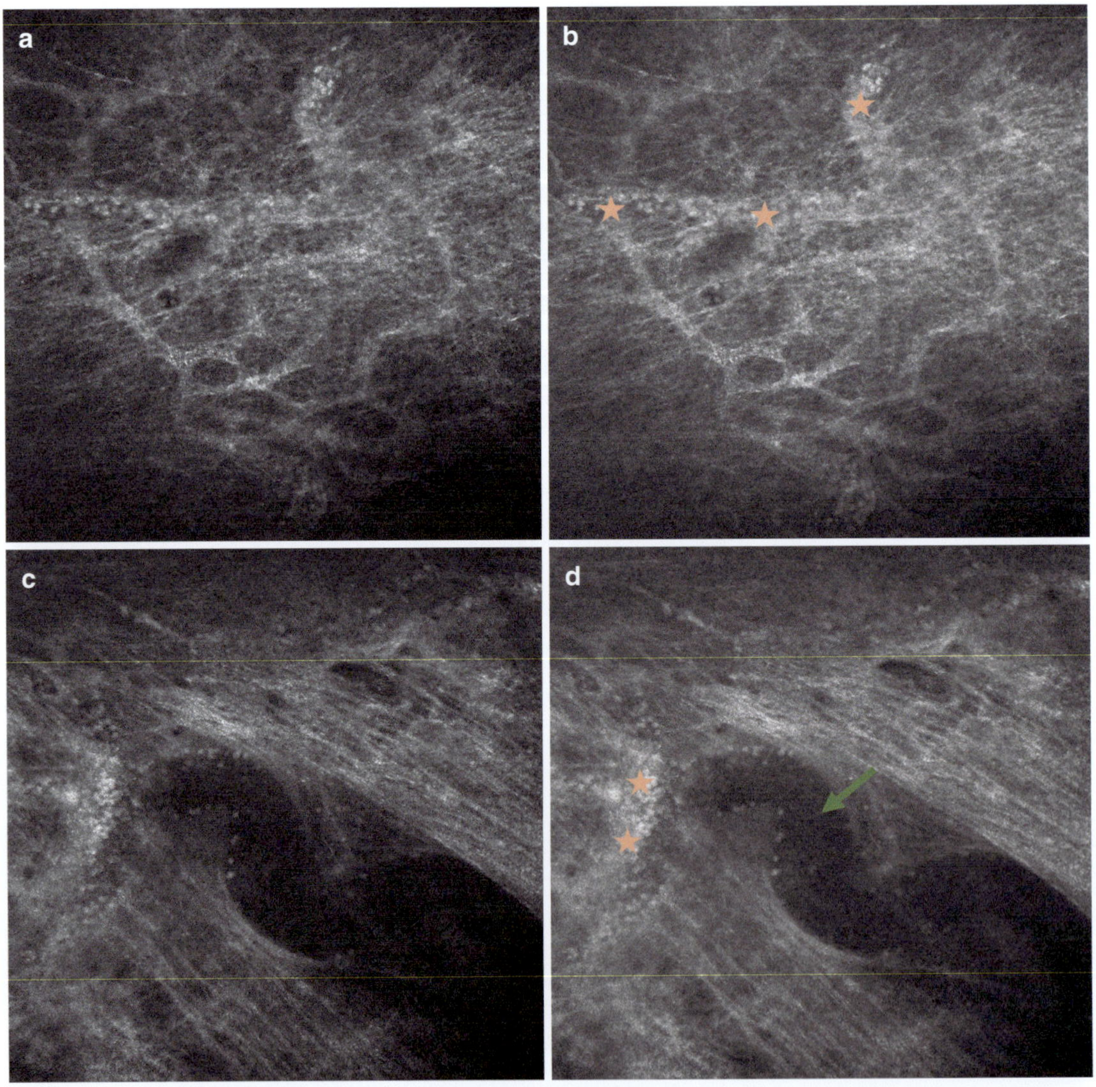

Fig. 15.11 IVCM features of mucosa-associated lymphoid tissue (**a**–**d**)

– Disorganized chorion containing small hyper-reflective roundish cells (*orange stars*) corresponding to tumor lymphocytes
– Dilated and tortuous vessels (*green arrow*)

On optical microscopy the histologic features are as follows (Fig. 15.12e–i):

– At low magnification (e, f), a proliferation of small monomorphic lymphocytes (*orange stars*) in the chorion
– The immunohistochemistry study (g) shows that this proliferation is marked by the anti-CD20 antibody in brown (g.1) and by the anti-PAX5 antibody in brown (g.2). In addition,

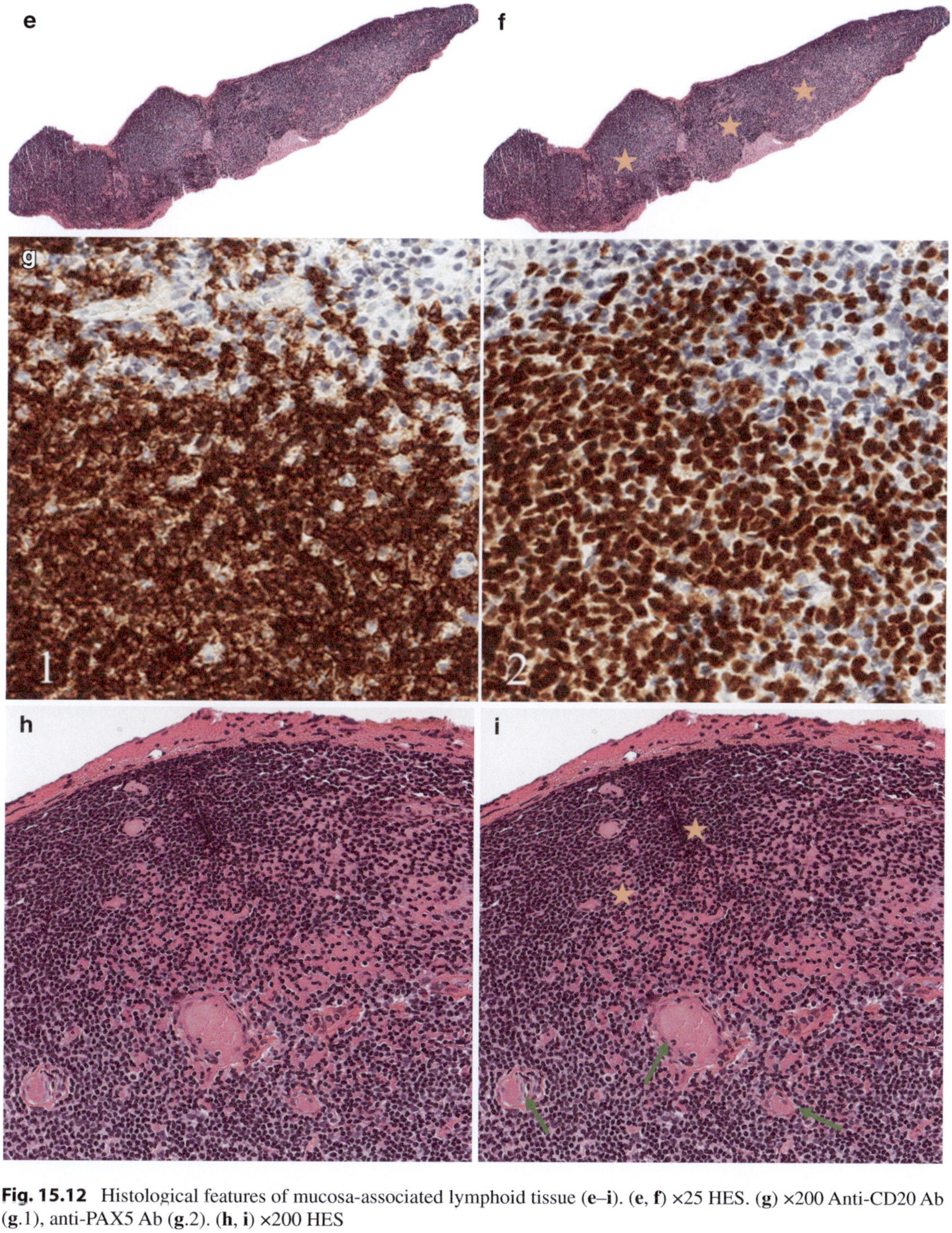

Fig. 15.12 Histological features of mucosa-associated lymphoid tissue (**e**–**i**). (**e**, **f**) ×25 HES. (**g**) ×200 Anti-CD20 Ab (**g**.1), anti-PAX5 Ab (**g**.2). (**h**, **i**) ×200 HES

there is no immunoreactivity to antibodies against CD5, CD10, CD23, and cycline D1.

- At high magnification (h, i), the architecture is in clusters and composed of small- to medium-sized lymphocytes (*orange stars*). No mitotic figures are observed. The connective tissue is richly vascularized (*green arrows*).

MIX
Papier aus verantwortungsvollen Quellen
Paper from responsible sources
FSC® C105338

If you have any concerns about our products,
you can contact us on
ProductSafety@springernature.com

In case Publisher is established outside the EU,
the EU authorized representative is:
Springer Nature Customer Service Center GmbH
Europaplatz 3, 69115 Heidelberg, Germany

Printed by Libri Plureos GmbH
in Hamburg, Germany